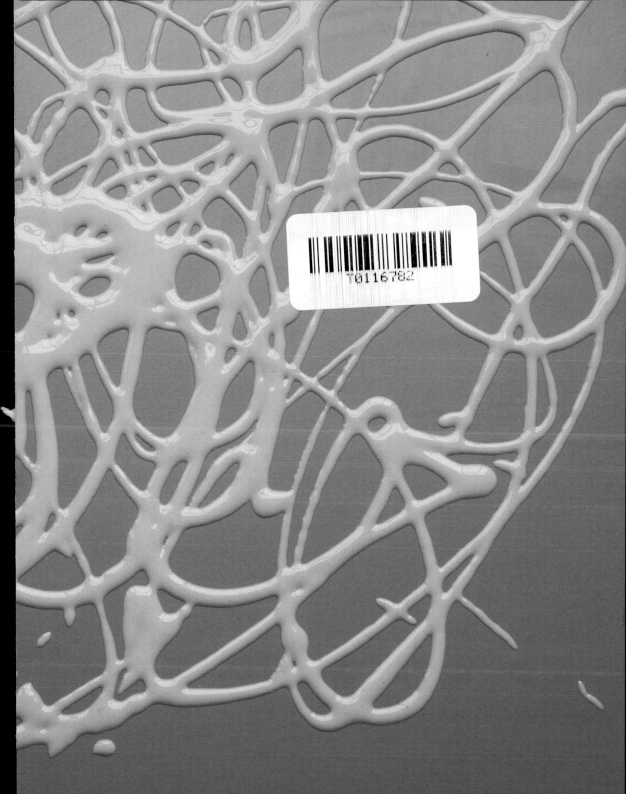

THE MAGIC OF
TAHINI

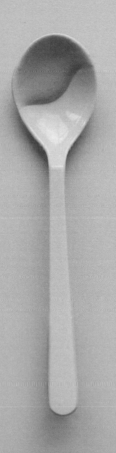

THE MAGIC OF
TAHINI

DUNJA GULIN
PHOTOGRAPHY BY CLARE WINFIELD

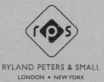

RYLAND PETERS & SMALL
LONDON • NEW YORK

DREAMY
VEGAN
RECIPES
ENRICHED
WITH SWEET
& NUTTY
SESAME
SEED PASTE

Senior designer Megan Smith
Editor Miriam Catley
Production Mai-Ling Collyer
Art director Leslie Harrington
Editorial director Julia Charles
Publisher Cindy Richards

Food stylist Emily Kydd
Prop stylist Alexander Breeze
Indexer Vanessa Bird

First published in 2019 by
Ryland Peters & Small
20–21 Jockey's Fields,
London WC1R 4BW
and 341 E 116th St, New York
NY 10029
www.rylandpeters.com

10 9 8 7 6 5 4 3 2 1

Text copyright © Dunja Gulin 2019
Design and photographs
copyright
© Ryland Peters & Small 2019

ISBN: 978-1-78879-072-7

Printed in China

A CIP record for this book
is available from the British
Library. US Library of Congress
Cataloging-in-Publication Data
has been applied for.

NOTES

• Both British (Metric) and
American (Imperial plus US
cups) measurements are
included in these recipes for
your convenience, however it is
important to work with one set
of measurements only and not
alternate between the two within
a recipe.
• All spoon measurements are
level unless otherwise specified.
A teaspoon is 5 ml, a tablespoon
is 15 ml.
• When a recipe calls for grated
zest of citrus fruit, buy unwaxed
organic fruit and wash well
before using. If you can only find
treated fruit, scrub well in warm
soapy water before using.
• Ovens should be preheated
to the specified temperatures.
We recommend using an
oven thermometer. If using
a fan-assisted oven, adjust
temperatures according to the
manufacturer's instructions.

CONTENTS

TAHINI
101

SESAME SEEDS are the key ingredient in tahini. These tiny, flat oval seeds come in a variety of colours including white, yellow, black and red. Sesame seed plants have been grown in tropical regions around the world since prehistoric times. They are considered to be the oldest oilseed crop known to mankind and are referenced in ancient Hindu legends, representing immortality.

The cultivated sesame crop is thought to have originated in India, and was then introduced to Africa, the Middle East, Asia and later, during the late 17th century, to the United States. Today, the largest producers are found in India, China and Mexico.

These tiny yet powerful seeds are more valuable to our diets than you might think. They are rich in beneficial minerals: an excellent source of copper and manganese and a good source of calcium, magnesium, iron, phosphorus, vitamin B1, zinc, molybdenum and selenium. They also contain sesamin and sesamolin – both shown to have a cholesterol-lowering effect in humans.

Among their many nutritional benefits, sesame seeds are often cited as being a great source of calcium for vegans; however, there is some controversy surrounding this topic. Hulled sesame seeds contain around 60% less calcium than sesame seeds with the hulls left intact. With this in mind, it makes sense that those who choose to eat a diet rich in unprocessed, wholesome foods (myself included!) will opt to purchase and consume the unhulled seeds, as well as tahini made from them. However, the type of calcium found in the hulls of sesame seeds is in the form of calcium oxalate – a different and less absorbable type of calcium than the calcium found in the kernels themselves. Therefore, we won't necessarily be consuming the full 60% more calcium if we choose to eat unhulled sesame seeds. It is likely, though, that we will absorb a bit more calcium overall from sesame seeds that contain the hulls, and don't forget that it's not just about the calcium – unhulled seeds are far richer in other nutrients as well.

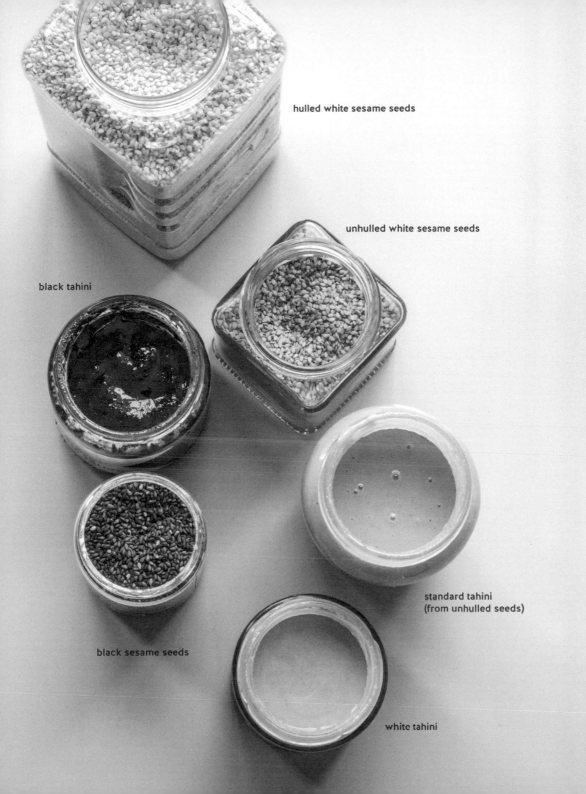

hulled white sesame seeds

unhulled white sesame seeds

black tahini

standard tahini
(from unhulled seeds)

black sesame seeds

white tahini

TYPES OF TAHINI
& HOW THEY'RE MADE

Types of tahini paste vary in taste and texture, depending on how the original ingredient is processed. Tahinis made from the hulled variety of sesame seeds are creamier and taste less bitter than those made with the unhulled seeds.

Both hulled and unhulled seeds can then be used raw, lightly toasted or dark toasted to make tahini. In general, raw seeds give a more bitter taste and make tahini with a thicker consistency, whereas toasting the seeds tends to make tahini with a smoother texture and sweeter taste.

Commercially-made traditional tahini is produced from soaked and hulled sesame seeds, which are then toasted and ground. This process results in a smooth paste that is less bitter than the tahini made from unhulled seeds – it tastes slightly sweet and is therefore suitable for using in all types of recipes, from soups to desserts, without the risk of overpowering other flavours.

In this cookbook, whenever a recipe calls for this mild, commercial variety of tahini, you will see 'white tahini' stated on the ingredients list. However, the tahini I use most often is homemade using organic, unhulled, lightly-toasted sesame seeds. It's the most nutritious option, since you can control the entire process and exactly what goes in. I use freshly toasted seeds to make small batches of tahini that will keep for up to a month. I don't add anything else to my tahini – no oil or salt – but you need to have a high-speed blender in order to achieve a really creamy consistency. If you are using a less powerful blender, you will mostly likely need to add a little oil to help the blending process.

If you don't have the time or proper equipment to make your own tahini, buying organic, lightly toasted tahini made from hulled seeds or organic lightly toasted tahini made from unhulled sesame seeds are the next best options. Different types of tahini can usually be found in health food stores or ethnic grocery stores throughout the world.

Store-bought black tahini is also available for interesting desserts such as Black Tahini & Poppy Seed Swirls (see page 95) and Black Tahini and Coconut Ice Cream (see page 111).

STORING TAHINI

The oil found in sesame seeds is highly resistant to rancidity, you just need to follow these simple guidelines to ensure your jar of tahini stays fresh:

* Keep it in a tightly covered glass container.
* Do not lick or wet the spoon you'll be using, just a little water can easily spoil the whole jar.
* Most tahinis can be stored for months at room temperature, but manufacturers of raw tahini recommend refrigeration to prevent spoilage. If you don't think you will use up your tahini within two months, keep it refrigerated, especially in summer.
* When tahini is sitting for a while, the oil and the solids might separate. This is totally fine and does not affect the quality of the tahini, just stir well before using!

HOW TO USE TAHINI

Most people buy a jar of tahini and use it in only a couple of well known recipes such as hummus, maybe a dressing and an occasional smoothie. In this book, my intention is to show you how to use it almost every day in all kinds of recipes.

Adding tahini to smoothies, soups, sauces and dressings boosts their nutritional value, improves the taste and slightly thickens the texture. As well as the healthy snacks, treats, baking and desserts, many different savoury main and side dishes can also be enriched with tahini. Its texture can be a great substitute in recipes that call for oil, and it's also a great substitute for peanut butter, if you are allergic to peanuts or just want to experiment a bit.

During my pregnancy, I was determined to eat at least two spoonfuls of tahini every day in order to increase my calcium intake, and most of the recipes offered in this cookbook are the direct result of my personal mission to discover all kinds of ways to sneak tahini into my diet and not get bored with it!

I sincerely hope that these recipes will inspire you to use tahini in new and unique ways, and encourage you to make it at home from scratch – what better way to improve your diet than by enjoying healthful, delicious food made with tahini. Enjoy!

HOMEMADE TAHINI

**260 g/2 cups unhulled
  sesame seeds
2 tablespoons oil (optional)**

MAKES ABOUT 260 G/1 CUP TAHINI

Put the sesame seeds into a fine-mesh sieve/ strainer and wash under cold running water, mixing with a spoon to make sure all the sesame seeds are wet. As well as removing any dust from the seeds, this step will ensure that the seeds toast evenly and will prevent them from jumping out of the hot pan. Drain the seeds well.

Transfer the drained seeds to a dry frying pan/skillet over a medium heat and, using a wooden spoon, stir continuously until all the moisture has evaporated.

Once the seeds are dry, continue to stir vigorously and continuously, making sure the seeds are always on the move to prevent them from burning. This stage needs your full attention and is a great test of patience. The entire toasting process takes about 10 minutes. The trickiest part is knowing when the seeds are toasted properly. Unevenly cooked seeds will result in a bitter tahini, which is also true for seeds that have been over-toasted and become dark brown in colour. The key is to toast the seeds until they become fragrant, are lightly coloured and the majority of them have puffed up with a small popping sound. A good test is to take a few seeds between your fingers and pinch them – if they are ready they should easily crush into a powder.

Transfer the toasted seeds to a dry bowl or plate to cool slightly, then place in a high-speed blender and blend on low speed, pushing the seeds with the blender tamper to make sure they are constantly on the move. Gradually increase the speed. The seeds should first turn into flour and then start releasing the oil. After a couple of minutes, you should get a smooth oily paste; your homemade tahini!

If you are using a less powerful blender or a food processor fitted with an S-blade, you will need to add two tablespoons of light sesame oil at a time at the powder stage to help the blending process, until you get a thick, fairly smooth paste.

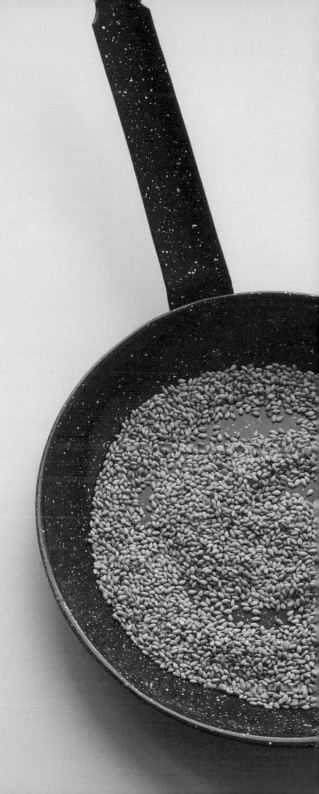

Transfer the tahini to a jar and leave uncovered until completely cool. Cover tightly and store at room temperature for up to 2 months or refrigerate for up to 6 months.

TO MAKE WHITE TAHINI
Use hulled sesame seeds and follow the instructions on page 10. Be careful when toasting, as sesame kernels toast faster and burn much more easy than unhulled seeds!

TO MAKE BLACK TAHINI
Follow the instructions on page 10 using the same amount of black sesame seeds. It will be slightly more difficult to tell when the seeds are ready because of their dark colour, so use the pinching method to test if they're ready.

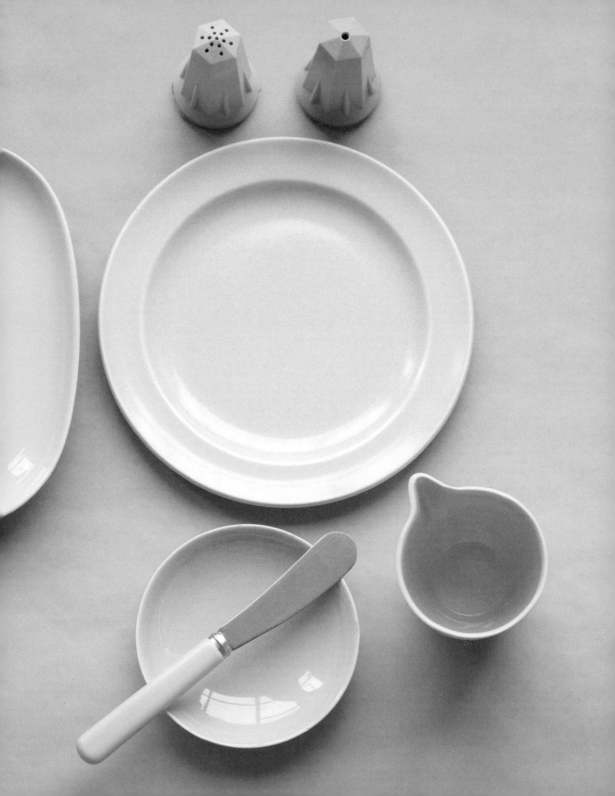

SNACKS & SOUPS

TAHINI POPCORN

I can safely say popcorn is the most popular snack in our household — we make it five days a week for sure! When we get bored with the plain, salted popcorn, I add different things to it to make it more interesting, and tahini popcorn is one of the best received variations.

4 tablespoons high-oleic sunflower oil
100 g/½ cup organic popcorn kernels
4 tablespoons tahini
1 tablespoon agave or maple syrup
salt, to taste

SERVES 2

Put the oil and popcorn kernels in a good-quality pot or pan with a tight-fitting lid. Place over a high heat and leave to pop, covered. Remove from the heat as soon as the popping stops.

In a small saucepan, whisk together the tahini and syrup over a low heat until melted.

Transfer the hot popcorn into a big serving bowl and drizzle with the tahini mix. Toss well to coat. Sprinkle with salt to taste and serve.

It's important to make a fresh batch each time you crave this delicious and nutritious snack, as leftovers (if there ever are any!) become somewhat soggy.

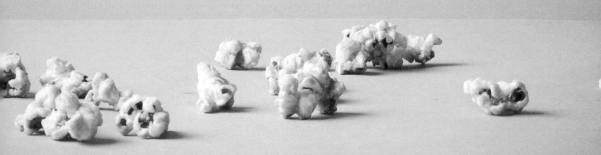

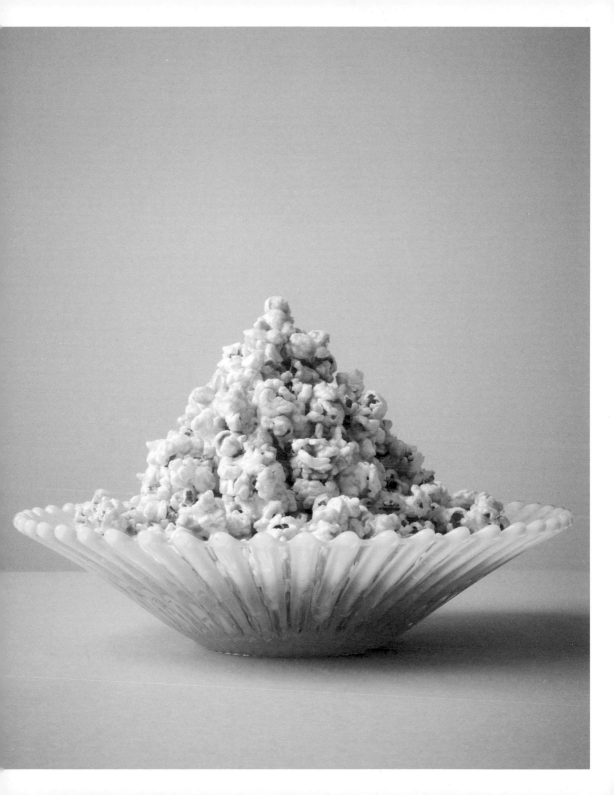

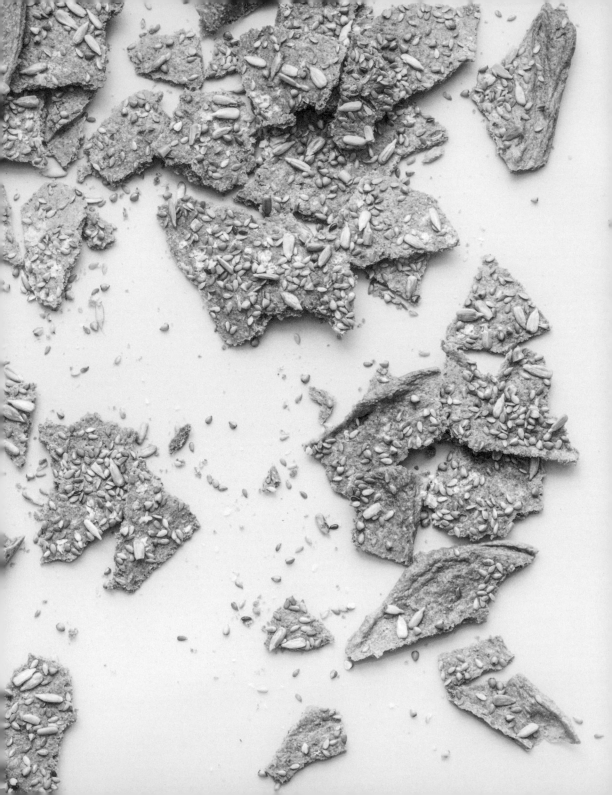

BUCKWHEAT & TAHINI CRACKERS

Gluten-free crackers are great to have on hand if you want to avoid eating a lot of bread or store-bought crackers. I always have a stash in my cupboard and make a double amount since they keep for over a month, if dried/baked well.

80 g/⅓ cup tahini
90 g/½ cup buckwheat
90 g/⅔ cup sunflower seeds, plus extra, for sprinkling (optional)
100 g/1 cup grated celery
¾ teaspoon salt
1 green (bell) pepper, deseeded
2 spring onions/scallions
2 tablespoons ground flaxseeds/linseeds
1 teaspoon flaxseeds/linseeds, for sprinkling (optional)
110 ml/⅓ cup plus 2 tablespoons celery juice or water

MAKES 20–24 CRACKERS

Preheat the oven to 80°C (175°F) or the very lowest gas setting.

In a high-speed blender blend all the ingredients into a thick paste. Cut a piece of baking parchment into the size of your oven rack/baking pan and place it on a smooth surface (kitchen counter or table). Spoon the cracker paste onto the baking parchment and spread very thinly into a rectangular shape with an even surface. Put the oven rack/baking pan on the edge of the counter and quickly pull the baking parchment to slide onto it. Sprinkle the paste with the extra sunflower seeds and the flaxseeds/linseeds, if using.

Place in the upper part of the preheated oven and increase the temperature to 100°C (225°F) Gas ¼. Prop the oven door open with a folded tea/dish towel, to ensure proper dehydration. Dehydrate for 2–3 hours.

Remove from the oven and peel off the baking parchment. Use a pizza cutter to cut into desired shapes or break into pieces, then return the crackers to the oven and dehydrate directly on the oven rack/baking pan for another 30 minutes if you want them totally crispy. I love them a bit on the soft side, but dry crackers last longer without spoiling. Use instead of bread or as a really healthy snack.

WALNUT TAHINI HUMMUS

A great take-away snack or a quick lunch, paired with homemade crackers, rice cakes or freshly baked bread, and a side salad.

200 g/1¼ cups walnuts, soaked for at least 4 hours and well drained, plus extra (chopped), to serve
80 g/⅓ cup tahini
60 ml/¼ cup extra virgin olive oil, plus extra to serve
60 ml/¼ cup freshly squeezed lemon juice, or to taste
¾ teaspoon salt, or to taste
1½ teaspoons crushed cumin seeds or 1 teaspoon ground cumin
2 garlic cloves, peeled
freshly ground black pepper
freshly chopped parsley, to serve

MAKES 370 G/1½ CUPS

In a food processor fitted with an 'S' blade or in a high-speed blender, blend all the ingredients together, adding 120 ml/1 cup water until you reach a creamy texture. Taste and adjust the seasoning.

Serve drizzled with a little extra olive oil and scattered with chopped walnuts and chopped herbs.

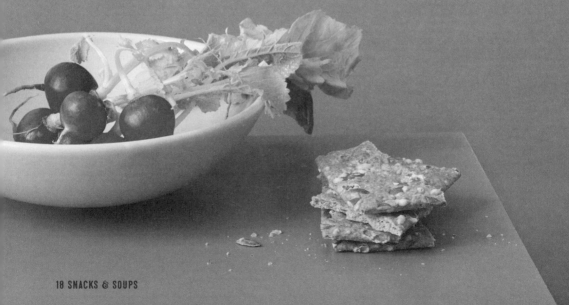

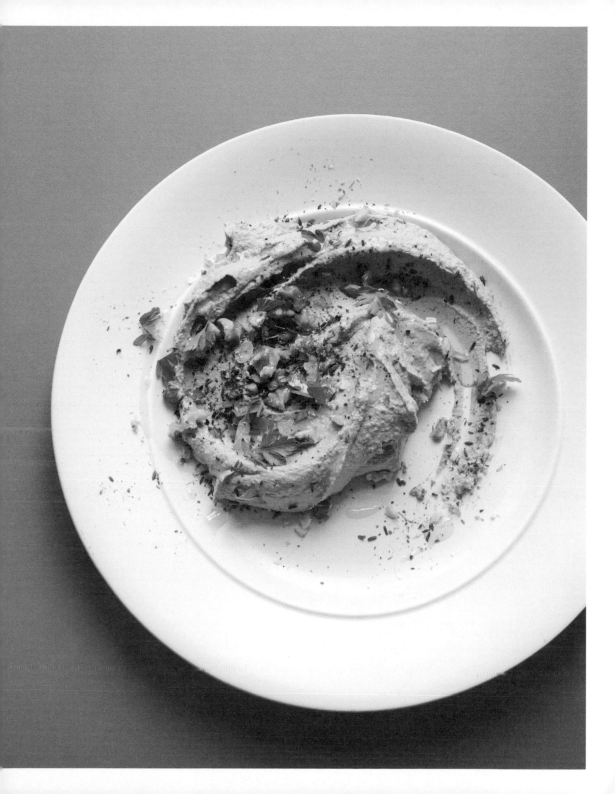

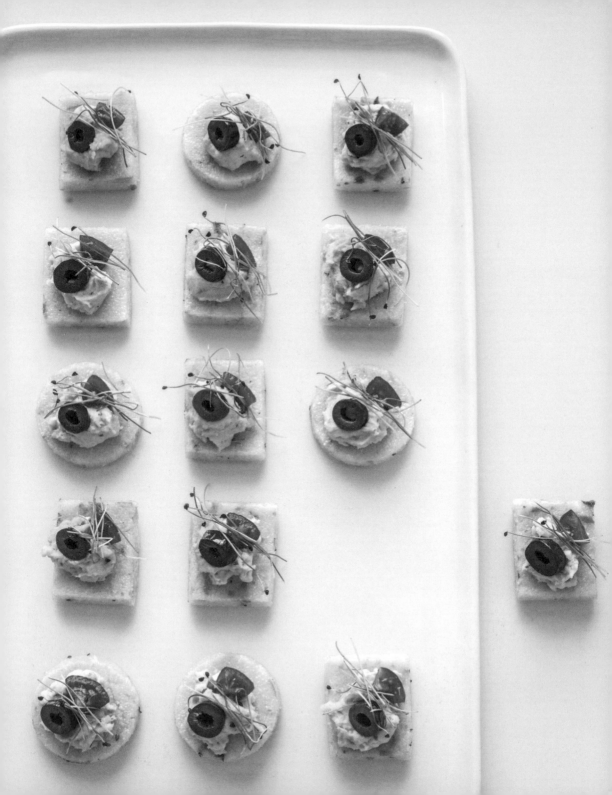

POLENTA CANAPÉS

Polenta/cornmeal, is such a simple, rustic ingredient that has been re-discovered recently, especially with the gluten-free movement becoming more global. It was a staple food for my Istrian grandparents and I really love its taste and texture, whether it's served as a porridge, a side dish or, as in this recipe, as a canapé base.

FOR THE BASE
90 g/½ cup polenta/cornmeal
¼ teaspoon salt
50 g/⅓ cup smoked tofu,
   finely grated, divided
a little olive oil, for oiling
   and drizzling

FOR THE BEAN & TAHINI PÂTÉ
160 g/1 cup cooked unsalted
   haricot/navy beans, well
   drained
60 g/¼ cup tahini
3 garlic cloves, peeled
1 tablespoon nutritional yeast
   (optional)
½ teaspoon salt, or to taste
2 tablespoons olive oil
¼ teaspoon dried oregano
crushed black pepper

TO SERVE
cherry tomatoes, chopped
pitted black olives, halved
snipped chives

23 x 30 cm/9 x 12 inch
   baking pan

MAKES 24

For the base, in a heavy-bottomed saucepan, bring 360 ml/1½ cups water to the boil and whisk in the polenta/cornmeal and salt. Cover, lower the heat to minimum and simmer for 10 minutes. Stir, add the grated tofu, remove from the heat and let it stand for 10 minutes, covered.

Oil the baking pan and spoon in the cooked polenta/cornmeal, spreading it into an even layer. Drizzle with a little oil and smooth out with a spatula. Leave to cool completely, then cut into small squares or use a well-oiled round cookie cutter to cut out circles.

For the pâté, blend the beans and tahini with the other ingredients into a chunky pâté. Taste and adjust the seasoning.

To assemble the canapés, lay out the polenta/cornmeal pieces on a plate or serving tray. Using two teaspoons, top each bite with a teaspoon of pâté, then top with a small piece of cherry tomato, half a black olive and a few snipped chives. These canapés can be made in advance as the polenta/cornmeal base does not get soggy as quickly as bread or crackers.

RYE & TAHINI CRACKERS

It's so quick and easy to make crackers that I sometimes wonder why people buy them. I've reduced the quantity of salt in my crackers to a minimum, since I usually serve them with some kind of spicy spread or dip, but if you plan to eat them as a snack, you can add more salt to the dough.

130 g/1 cup rye flour
130 g/1 cup unbleached plain/
   all-purpose flour
2 tablespoons black or unhulled
   sesame seeds
½ teaspoon salt
freshly ground black pepper
60 g/¼ cup tahini
1 teaspoon brown rice syrup

*baking sheet, lined with baking
   parchment*

MAKES ABOUT 16

Mix together the flours, seeds, salt and some pepper in a bowl. In a separate bowl, whisk the tahini and syrup with 60 ml/¼ cup water to emulsify. Slowly pour into the bowl of dry ingredients, stirring until well combined. The dough should quickly form a ball and shouldn't be sticky. Knead a couple of times, just enough to make sure all the ingredients are evenly distributed. Wrap the dough in clingfilm/plastic wrap and allow to rest at room temperature for 10 minutes. This will make rolling out the dough much easier. Divide the dough into three equal portions. Preheat the oven to 200°C (400°F) Gas 6.

Place the dough between sheets of baking parchment and use a rolling pin to roll it out very thinly. For really crunchy crackers, the dough should be almost paper-thin, but if you like a bit of texture, roll it to your preferred thickness. Use a knife or a pizza cutter to cut out shapes; squares or rectangles are most practical, as you'll have hardly any leftover dough. Re-roll any trimmings. Transfer the crackers to the prepared baking sheet using a spatula or thin knife. Prick each one a couple of times with a fork

Bake in the preheated oven for 4–7 minutes, depending on the thickness of the crackers. Remember that they shouldn't brown, just get slightly golden. They will firm up as they cool, so don't expect them to be cracker-crunchy straight out of the oven! Allow to cool completely and store in an airtight container for 1–2 weeks.

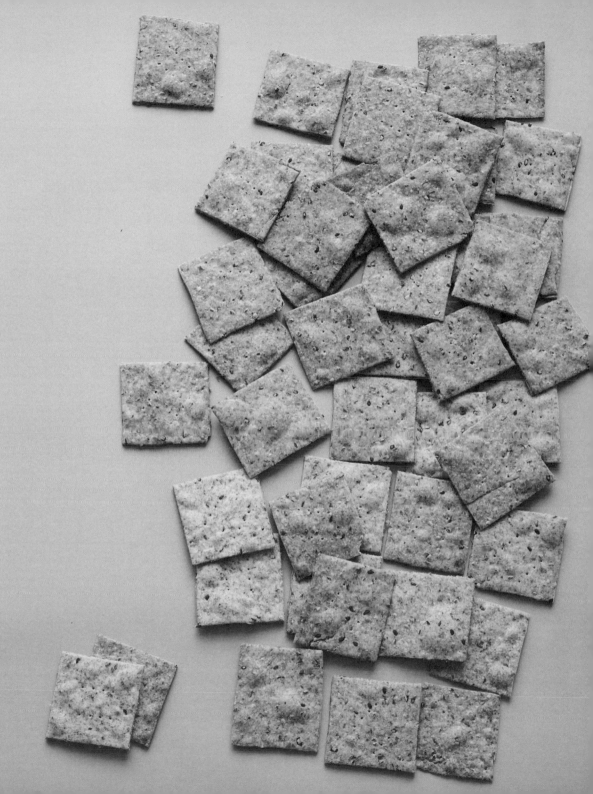

TAHINI 'CHEESE' NACHOS

A typical Tex-Mex snack: fried tortilla chips served with nacho 'cheese'— in this case with a healthy vegan twist!

1 carrot or 1 slice of pumpkin
   (approx. 100 g/3½ oz. peeled,
   deseeded and cut into cubes)
60 g/½ cup chopped onion
220 g/1 cup silken tofu
2 tablespoons white tahini
1 tablespoon umeboshi vinegar
   or apple cider vinegar
1 tablespoon nutritional yeast
½ teaspoon smoked paprika
½ teaspoon chilli/chili powder
1 garlic clove, peeled
2 tablespoons sunflower oil
½ teaspoon salt, or to taste
freshly squeezed lemon juice,
   to taste
tortilla chips or crunchy
   vegetables, to serve

MAKES 360 ML/1½ CUPS

Blanch the carrot or pumpkin in a little boiling water or steam, until soft. Blend all the ingredients into a smooth 'cheese' sauce. Taste and adjust the seasoning.

Pour over tortilla chips or crunchy vegetables, as an appetizer starter or a snack. This 'cheese' can also be served as a party dip, and it tastes even better if left to rest in the fridge overnight.

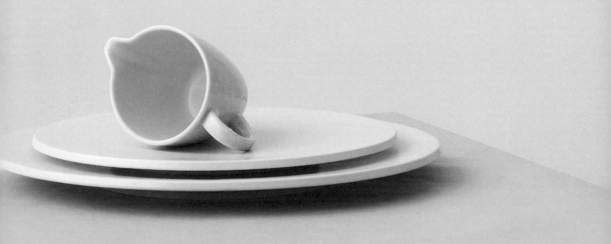

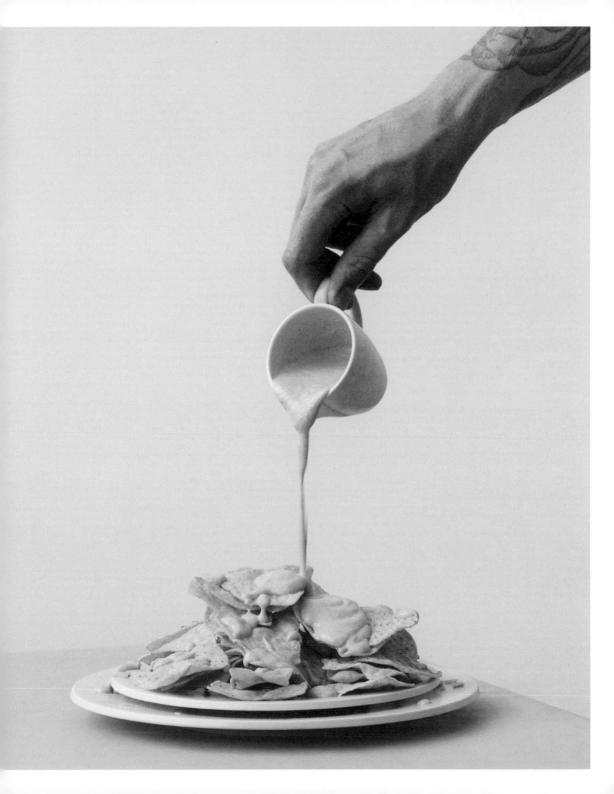

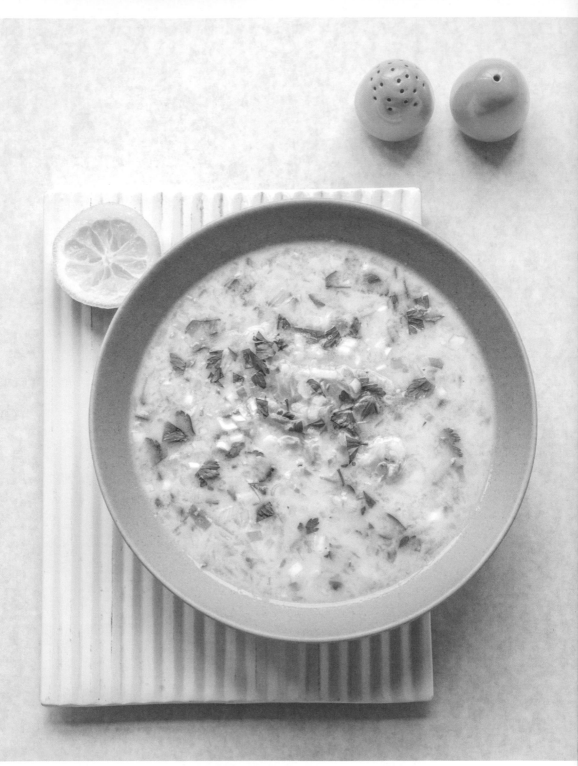

GREEK TAHINIOSOUPA WITH RICE

During my prolonged stay in Greece, I enjoyed a soup similar to this one, served for dinner at room temperature on hot summer evenings. Traditionally, miniature pasta is used, but I prefer the taste and texture of rice, especially if the soup sits for a day and the rice absorbs some of the liquid and gets really soft and creamy.

60 g/⅓ cup Arborio rice
70 g/1 celery stalk, grated
50 g/⅓ cup grated courgette/zucchini
2 teaspoons salt, or to taste
80 g/⅓ cup tahini, mixed well
2 tablespoons freshly chopped parsley
2 spring onions/scallions, finely chopped
freshly squeezed juice of 1 lemon, or to taste

SERVES 3-4

Bring 1.4 litres/6 cups water to the boil in a saucepan, add the rice and simmer for 7–8 minutes. Add the celery, courgette/zucchini and salt and simmer for another 5 minutes, then remove from the heat.

Dilute the tahini with a little hot broth and whisk into the soup. Cover and let it stand for 10 minutes.

Stir in the chopped parsley, spring onions/scallions and lemon juice, taste, adjust the seasoning and serve warm or at room temperature.

THAI SOUP WITH TAHINI & TOFU

So many people nowadays are allergic to peanuts, so when I cook for big groups I often substitute peanut butter with tahini, with great results! Tahini adds thickness, creaminess and taste to the stock and in combination with plenty of greens makes this soup super rich in calcium.

1 carrot
1 red (bell) pepper, deseeded
3 tablespoons virgin coconut oil
1 onion, chopped
3 tablespoons finely chopped (peeled) fresh ginger
160 g/1 cup cubed tofu
1 red chilli/chile, deseeded and thinly sliced, or ½ teaspoon chilli/chili powder
4 tablespoons tamari soy sauce, plus extra to taste
1.2 litres/5 cups boiling water
180 g/4 cups dried flat rice noodles
2–4 tablespoons tahini
2 tablespoons rice or apple cider vinegar
2 tablespoons agave syrup or demerara/turnbinado sugar
2 handfuls of greens (spinach, chard, kale, etc.), chopped
2 garlic cloves, thinly chopped
2 spring onions/scallions, finely sliced
2 teaspoons freshly squeezed lemon juice
4 tablespoons salted peanuts or cashews, chopped
salt

SERVES 2

Slice the carrot and red (bell) pepper into thick matchsticks. Heat the coconut oil in a heavy-bottomed saucepan and sauté the onion, carrot and (bell) pepper with the ginger, adding a pinch of salt. Add the tofu, chilli/chile slices or chilli/chili powder and tamari and cook until browned.

Add the boiling water and the dried rice noodles and bring to the boil. Whisk in the tahini, vinegar and syrup or sugar, stir well and cook over a medium heat for a couple of minutes. Add the chopped greens and cook for another minute or two, making sure the noodles do not overcook.

Remove from the heat and add the chopped garlic, spring onions/scallions, extra tamari, the lemon juice and salt to taste. Divide between two bowls, sprinkle with chopped nuts and dig in. Chopsticks and slurping are mandatory!

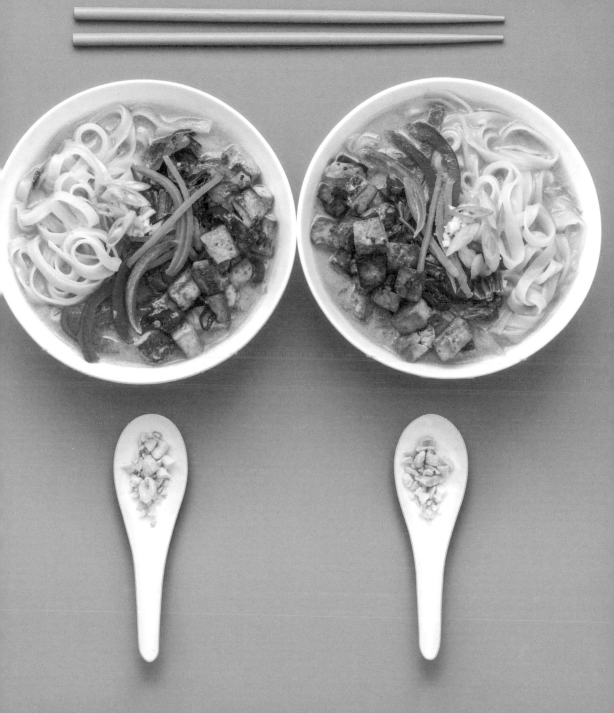

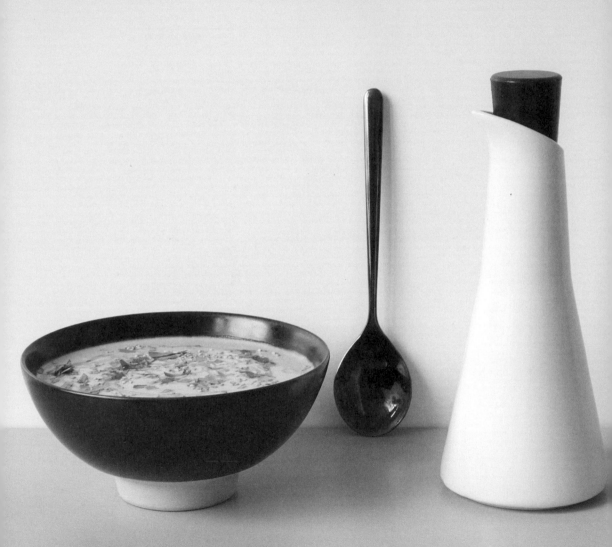

VELVETY MOCK MUSHROOM SOUP

I'm a big fan of creamy vegetable soups — you get to use up and eat a substantial amount of veggies in them and feed your family ingredients they might otherwise refuse to even taste. Cauliflower is definitely not everybody's cup of tea, but in this velvety soup it imitates the rich taste of mushrooms with the help of tahini and tamari soy sauce.

1 onion, chopped

2 garlic cloves, crushed

2 tablespoons light sesame oil, plus extra (optional) to serve

400 g/4 cups cauliflower florets

2 tablespoons tamari soy sauce

20 g/¼ cup fine rolled/porridge oats

60 g/¼ cup white tahini

salt and freshly ground black pepper

4 tablespoons snipped chives or other freshly chopped herbs, to serve

2 tablespoons toasted unhulled sesame seeds, to serve

SERVES 3-4

In a large pan, briefly sauté the onion and garlic in the sesame oil with a pinch of salt. Add the cauliflower and another pinch of salt and sauté for another couple of minutes. Add the tamari and stir well until it starts sticking to the bottom of the pan. Add the rolled oats and 960 ml/4 cups boiling water, then half-cover and simmer for 10–15 minutes, until the cauliflower becomes soft.

Add the tahini and salt to taste, then blend into a creamy soup using an immersion or high-speed blender, adding more hot water if necessary to reach the desired consistency. Season with black pepper.

Top each soup serving with snipped chives or chopped herbs and sprinkle with toasted sesame seeds. Add an extra drizzle of sesame oil if desired.

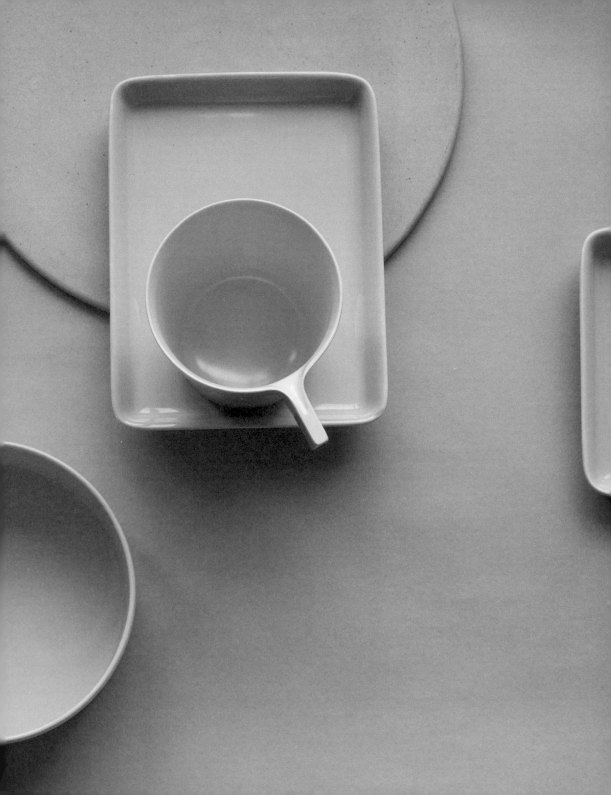

DRINKS & SWEET TREATS

PROTEIN SPIRULINA SHAKE

I have to admit I'm not a big fan of the taste of spirulina, but since it's such a healthy superfood, I try to use it from time to time in milkshakes, adding bananas and tahini to camouflage its seaweed flavour.

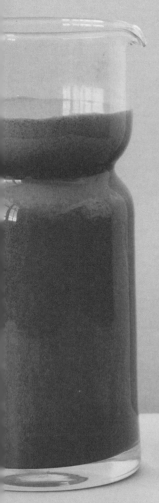

480 ml/2 cups soy milk, unsweetened
2 tablespoons tahini
1 tablespoon chia or flaxseeds/ linseeds
½–1 tablespoon spirulina powder
1–2 very ripe bananas, peeled
1 organic eating apple, peeled and cored
handful of baby spinach
1 teaspoon pure vanilla extract

SERVES 2

Blend all the ingredients into a creamy milkshake, adding a little water if the mixture is too thick. Pour into a glass to serve.

BEETROOT SMOOTHIE WITH TAHINI

The combination of beet juice and tahini might sound a bit off, but I assure you, you'll love this nutritious pink treat!

360 ml/1½ cups almond milk, or other plant-based milk
240 ml/1 cup beet(root) juice
4 tablespoons tahini
1 teaspoon pure vanilla extract
¼ teaspoon ground Ceylon cinnamon
4 tablespoons raisins or 4 soft pitted dates

SERVES 1–2

Blend all the ingredients into a creamy smoothie. Beet(root) juice can be substituted with ½ medium beet(root) and an additional 120 ml/½ cup water. If you don't own a high-speed blender, grate the raw beet(root) before blending. For a different colour and flavour, try using carrot, celery or mixed vegetable juice in place of beet(root) juice. Pour into a glass to serve.

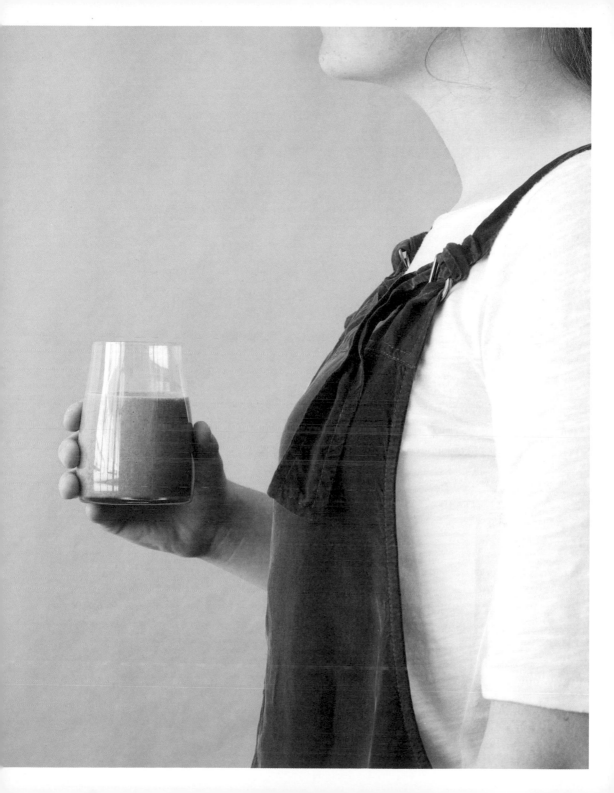

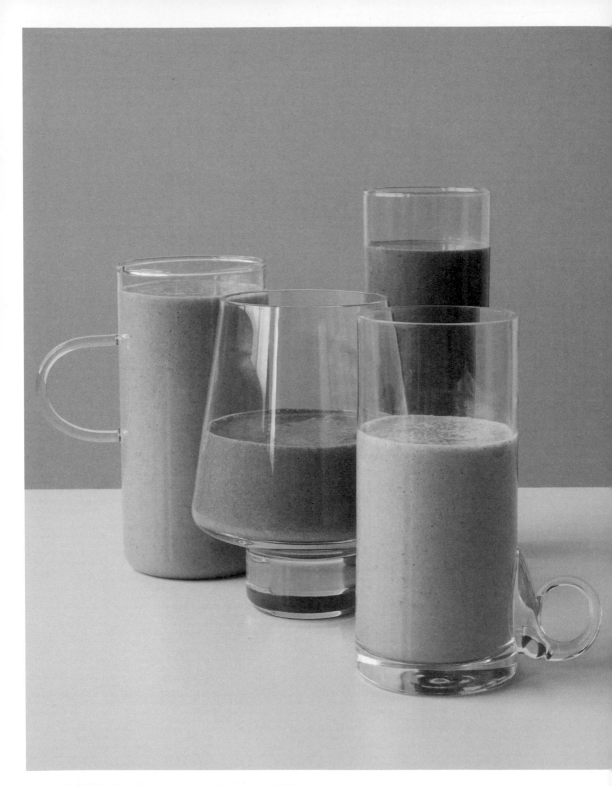

FRAPUCCINO

Yet another surprising and yummy combination of ingredients! This smoothie is quite filling and makes a great start to your day.

4 tablespoons buckwheat,
   pre-soaked
480 ml/2 cups almond milk,
   or other plant-based milk
3 tablespoons carob powder
2 tablespoons white tahini
70 g/1 piece of celeriac/
   celery root, peeled
¼ teaspoon ground Ceylon
   cinnamon
4 soft pitted dates, or to taste

SERVES 1–2

To soak the buckwheat, cover it with warm water and leave it to sit for 1 hour, or longer. Blend all the ingredients into a creamy smoothie. If you don't own a high-speed blender, grate the celeriac/celery root before blending. Carob powder can be substituted with raw cacao powder and buckwheat with fine rolled/porridge oats. Pour into glasses to serve.

COCONUT & STRAWBERRY FRAPPÉ

Strawberries are my favourite berries for smoothies, but you can substitute them with other fresh fruit — raspberries, blackberries, eating apples or ripe apricots also make a great combination with the nut milk and coconut water.

240 ml/1 cup raw organic
   coconut water
240 ml/1 cup unsweetened
   vanilla almond or oat milk
400 g/3 cups fresh strawberries
2 tablespoons white tahini
6 soft pitted dates, or to taste
few drops of freshly squeezed
   lemon juice

SERVES 2

Place all the ingredients in a blender and blend until completely smooth and foamy. Pour into glasses to serve. Drink immediately!

BLUEBERRY SMOOTHIE

Banana-blueberry is a classic combo. Adding tahini won't affect the taste, but as we all want to consume bioavailable calcium daily, add it every time!

480 ml/2 cups unsweetened vanilla almond or oat milk
220 g/1½ cups frozen blueberries
2 frozen bananas (flesh only)
60 g/¼ cup tahini
2 tablespoons flaxseeds/linseeds

SERVES 2

Blend all the ingredients in a high-speed blender until smooth and creamy. Add a little more milk, if necessary. Divide into two glasses and serve immediately.

CARAMEL SMOOTHIE

Full of goodness, this smoothie is a great way to sneak celeriac into your (and your kids') diet!

480 ml/2 cups coconut milk, or other plant-based milk
70 g/1 piece of celeriac/celery root, peeled
2 tablespoons tahini
1 tablespoon peanut butter, unsalted
1 teaspoon psyllium powder (optional)
1 teaspoon pure vanilla extract
4 soft pitted dates, or to taste

SERVES 1-2

Blend all the ingredients into a creamy smoothie. If you don't own a high-speed blender, grate the celeriac before blending. If you can't find celeriac, you can substitute it with celery stalk or kohlrabi.

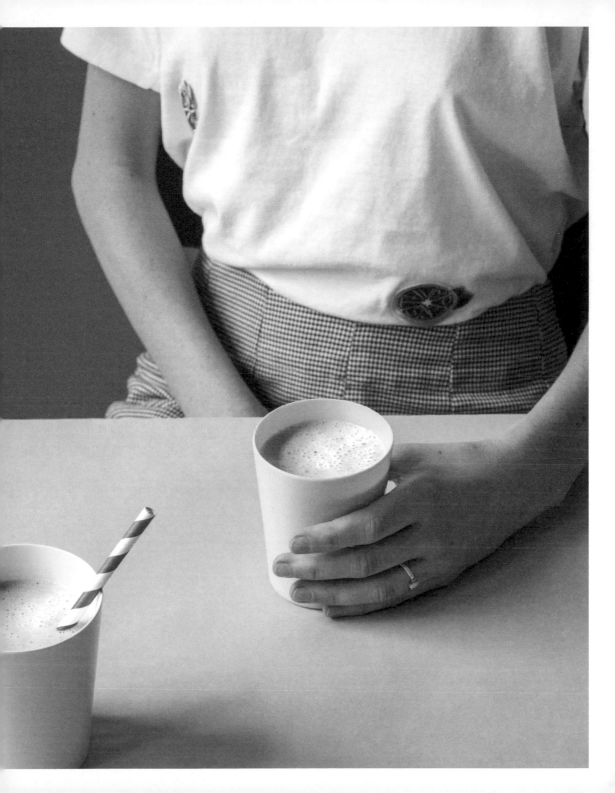

STRAWBERRY TAHINI 'YOGURT'

I don't think people consume strawberries as often as they should, so this is one of the ways to use them in (or out of) season. You can substitute with other milder-tasting berries like blueberries or raspberries, or even mix different berries in one batch.

160 ml/⅔ cup agave syrup
2 teaspoons agar agar powder or
   10 g/3½ tablespoons agar flakes
500 g/3 cups organic
   strawberries, fresh or frozen
330 g/1½ cups silken tofu
2 tablespoons white tahini
a few fresh strawberries,
   sliced or some strawberry
   jam/preserves, to decorate
   (optional)
edible flowers, to decorate
   (optional)

SERVES 4

In a small saucepan, whisk together the agave syrup and agar agar powder/flakes with 100 ml/⅓ cup plus 1 tablespoon water. Bring to the boil, whisking occasionally. If using agar flakes, simmer for about 5 minutes until the flakes have dissolved.

While the liquid is still hot, blend together the strawberries, silken tofu, tahini and cooked agar liquid. Pour into four serving cups or ramekins and chill well in the fridge before serving. If you wish, decorate with fresh strawberries or a dollop of strawberry jam/preserves, and edible flowers.

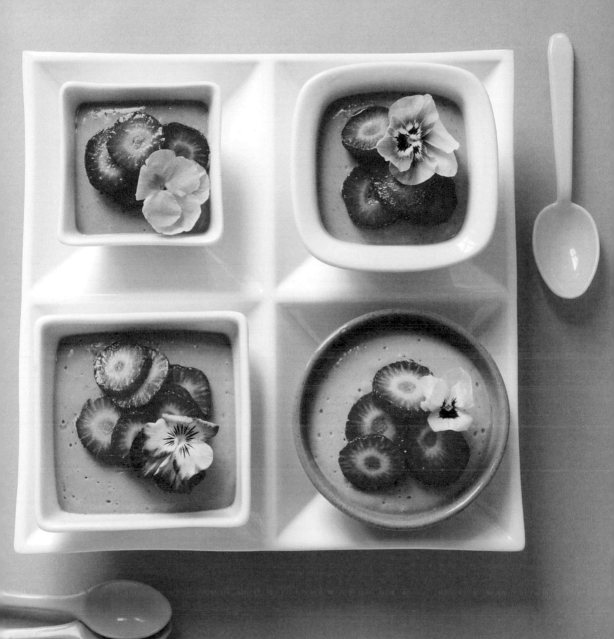

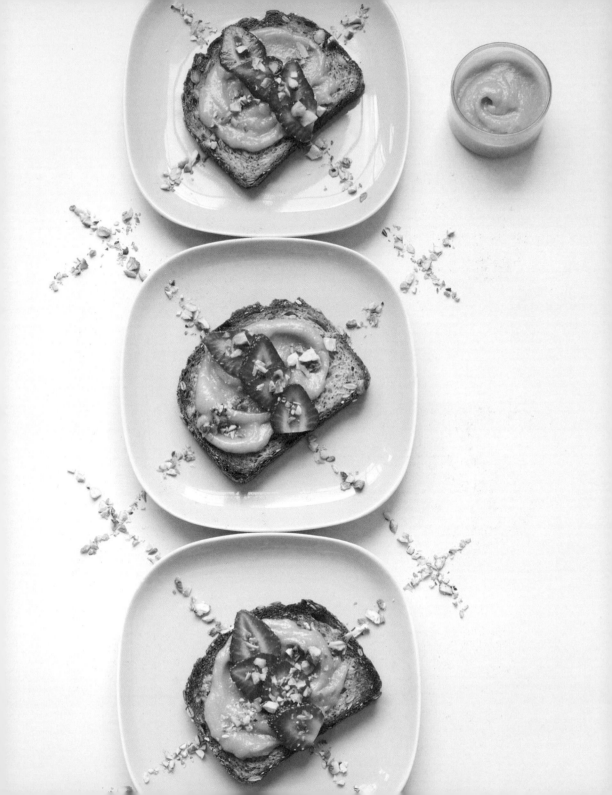

SWEET TAHINI 'BUTTER' SPREAD

If you love starting your day with toast, butter and jam, you have to try this!

4 tablespoons soy or oat cream
4 tablespoons white tahini
2–4 tablespoons rice or agave
  syrup
½ teaspoon pure vanilla extract
pinch of salt
4–5 slices of wholegrain bread,
  freshly toasted
4 tablespoons fruit jam/preserves
  or slices of fresh fruit, to serve

SERVES 2

In a small saucepan, slowly heat the cream to a gentle simmer, then remove from the heat and add the tahini, syrup, vanilla and salt. Whisk until smooth – the consistency should be thick enough to be easily spread over slices of toast.

Cover each slice of toast with the spread, then top with jam/preserves of your choice, sliced fresh fruit or any other topping you like (dried fruits, chopped nuts, etc.). Serve for breakfast or as an afternoon snack with a cup of hot grain coffee or tea.

NUTRITIOUS TAKE-AWAY BARS

There is always a stash of these bars in my fridge or freezer, each neatly wrapped up and ready to go! They are amazing for breakfast, as a pick-me-up snack or a guilt-free dessert. You can use millet flakes to make these bars gluten-free and any other dried fruits instead of apricots. Also, try adding orange zest and juice instead of lemon for the popular cacao-orange combo.

2 very ripe bananas
4 tablespoons tahini
15 unsulphured dried and diced apricots or prunes, or 40 g/⅓ cup raisins
grated zest of 1 organic lemon plus 1 tablespoon freshly squeezed lemon juice
1 teaspoon rum (optional)
200 g/2¼ cups fine rolled/porridge oats
¼ teaspoon ground Ceylon cinnamon
⅛ teaspoon bourbon vanilla powder
3 tablespoons raw cacao powder or carob powder
pinch of salt

18 x 18-cm/7 x 7-inch shallow dish or baking pan

MAKES 8 BARS

Peel the bananas and blend them with the tahini, dried fruits, lemon zest and juice and rum (if using) into a smooth paste. In a large bowl, combine the oats, cinnamon, vanilla powder, cocoa/carob and salt. Mix and add the banana paste to the dry ingredients. Use a spatula to combine the ingredients really well – there should be no dry patches of oats and the dough should be thick and sticky.

Line the base and sides of the dish or baking pan with clingfilm/plastic wrap. Place the dough in it and use a spatula or your hands to press down the mixture until you get an even layer about 1 cm/½ inch thick. Wrap well with more clingfilm/plastic wrap and freeze for an hour or longer.

Remove the clingfilm/plastic wrap and cut into 8 bars. Serve or wrap each one separately in baking parchment, keep in the freezer or fridge and eat within a week.

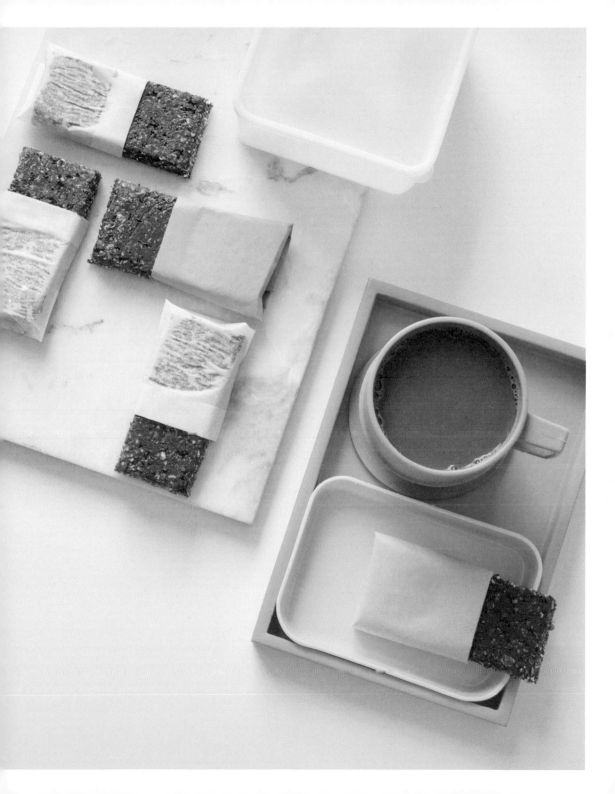

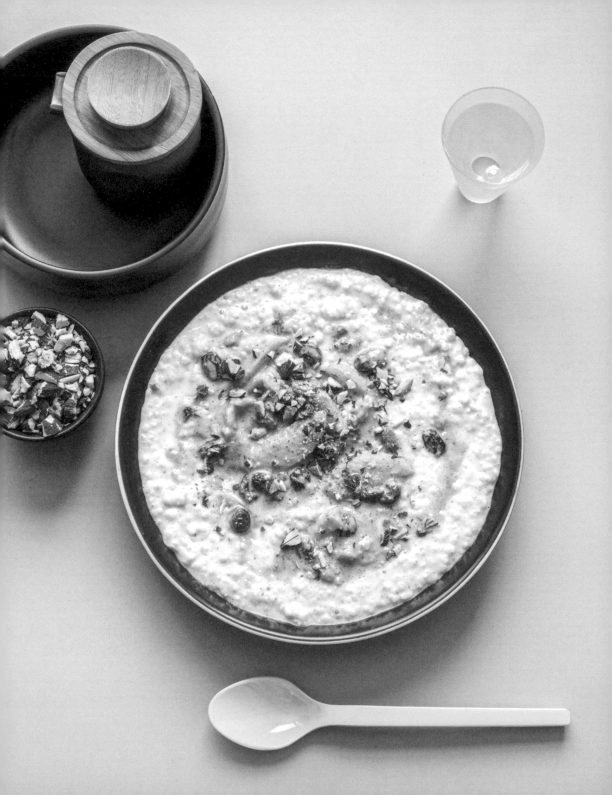

CREAMY PORRIDGE TOPPING

This porridge topping can be made in advance and reheated just before serving. My favourite porridge to go with this creamy recipe is soft millet porridge or soft brown rice porridge.

2 eating apples, peeled, cored and sliced
pinch of salt
240 ml/1 cup plant-based milk
30 g/¼ cup raisins or other dried fruit (optional)
60 g/¼ cup white tahini
¼ teaspoon ground Ceylon cinnamon
¼ teaspoon bourbon vanilla powder
4 tablespoons maple syrup
more hot milk or hot water, if needed
2 servings cooked soft millet or soft brown porridge
4 tablespoons roasted chopped almonds, to serve

SERVES 2

Place the apple slices in a saucepan, add the salt and milk (and dried fruits, if using) and simmer, covered, over a very low heat until the apples start to soften. Add the tahini, cinnamon, vanilla powder and syrup and stir well. If it's too thick, add a little more hot liquid.

Pour over hot porridge and enjoy! Sprinkle with chopped almonds, for an extra crunch.

CHIA HOT CHOCOLATE WITH TAHINI

I add chia seeds to my drinks and smoothies when I want them to be extra creamy. You can also soak them in water beforehand for better digestion and absorption of nutrients.

40 g/¼ cup unsalted cashews, soaked for at least 4 hours and drained
60 g/¼ cup tahini
2 tablespoons raw cacao powder
handful of young greens (spinach, chard, etc.)
3 soft pitted dates, or to taste
2 tablespoons chia seeds
pinch of ground Ceylon cinnamon
pinch of salt

SERVES 2

Blend all the ingredients with 480 ml/2 cups hot water until smooth. You can substitute the cashews and hot water with 480 ml/2 cups of any warmed plant-based milk, but in that case add another tablespoon of chia seeds to the mix to make the drink equally creamy. Pour into cups to serve.

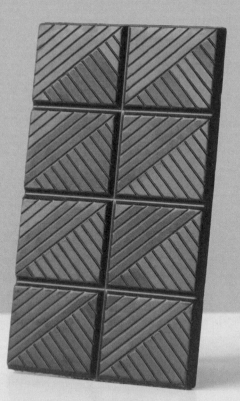

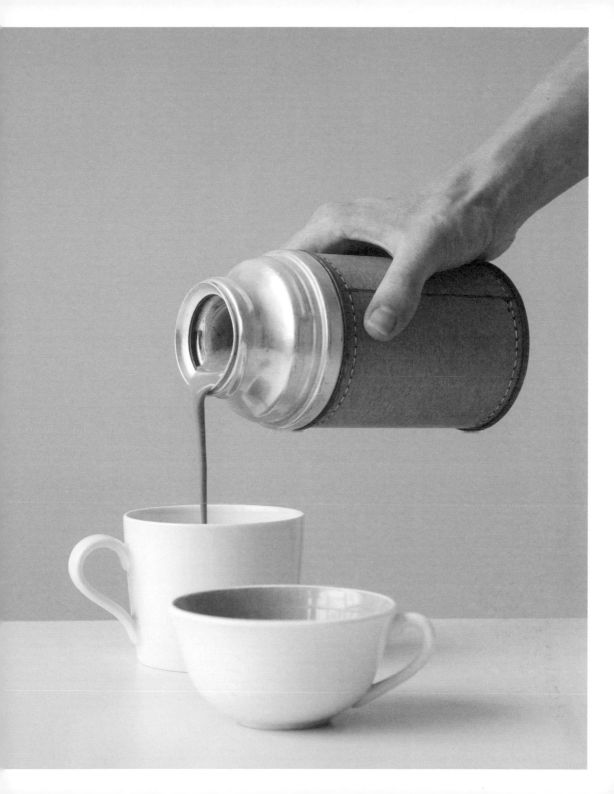

SWEET FENUGREEK & TAHINI BITES

Such an easy dessert to make, but it's even easier to eat the whole amount in one day, so hide them in the back of the freezer, just in case!

160 g/1 cup unsalted cashews or other nuts
40 g/¼ cup chia seeds
80 g/1 cup shredded coconut, divided
1 tablespoon ground fenugreek seeds
pinch of salt
180 g/1 cup Medjool dates, pitted
grated zest and freshly squeezed juice of 1 lemon, or to taste
130 g/½ cup tahini

MAKES ABOUT 30

Blend the nuts, chia seeds and half of the shredded coconut into fine flour and mix with the ground fenugreek and salt. Blend the dates with the lemon zest and juice separately and then add to the dry ingredients together with the tahini, and mix well. Knead well with moist hands, form into balls, then roll each ball in the remaining shredded coconut.

Freeze for 30 minutes before serving. Keep the leftovers in the freezer in an airtight container for up to 3 months and take them out 15 minutes before serving.

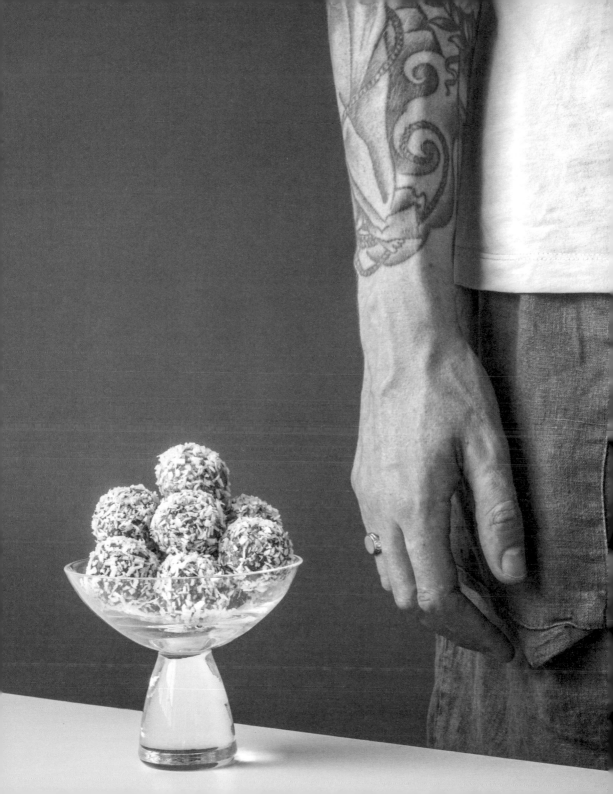

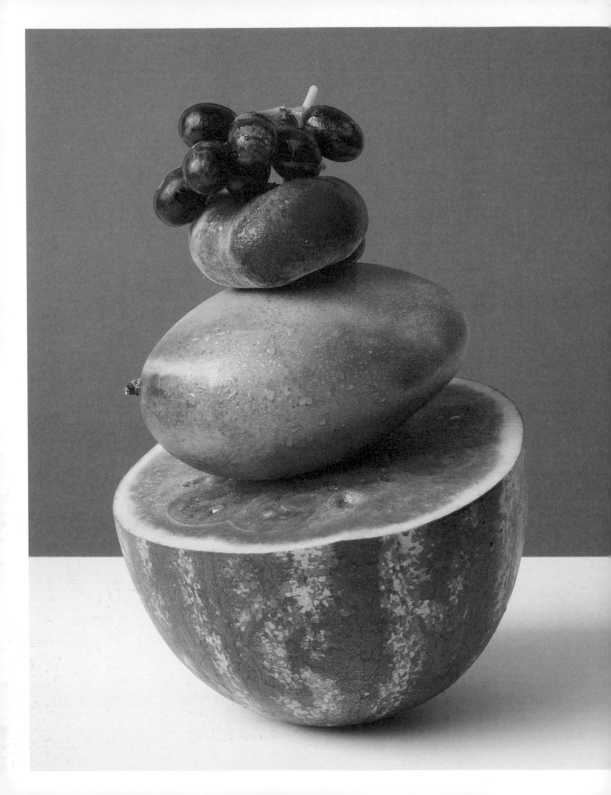

FRUIT KEBABS WITH CHOC-TAHINI DIP

A fun way to serve fresh fruit at both children's and adult parties. Why should party food always be unhealthy?

FOR THE DIP
260 g/1 cup tahini
130 ml/½ cup maple or date syrup
3 tablespoons raw cacao powder
1 teaspoon pure vanilla extract
plant-based milk, if needed

prepared fresh fruit (melon, pineapple, mango, grapes, apples, kiwi, strawberries, etc.), to serve

wooden skewers

MAKES 390 G/1½ CUPS

Mix together all the dip ingredients until smooth. If it's too thick, add a small amount of plant-based milk.

Cut the fruit into large pieces and thread alternately onto skewers. Arrange the fruit skewers on plates with some of the dip placed in a small bowl in the centre of each plate.

CREAMY TAHINI ICE LOLLIES

I love homemade ice cream, especially the kind that does not require an ice-cream maker! During hot summer days while I was pregnant, these lollies were my go-to treats. I was adding tahini to everything since it's rich in calcium, an important nutrient for mum and baby.

400-ml/14-oz. can coconut cream
2 ripe bananas, peeled
4 tablespoons tahini
2–4 tablespoons agave syrup
¼ teaspoon bourbon vanilla powder
2 tablespoons raw cacao nibs (optional)

6 ice-lolly/popsicle moulds and sticks

MAKES 6

Blend all the ingredients except the cacao nibs in a blender until creamy, then taste and adjust the sweetness, if needed. Fold in the nibs (if using). Fill the moulds, insert the sticks (if using) put on the lids and freeze for a couple of hours or overnight. To take the lollies out of the moulds, gently pass inside the edges with a sharp, wet knife, or quickly submerge each mould in hot water.

VARIATION Coconut cream can be substituted with full-fat coconut milk: refrigerate two 400-ml/14-oz. cans overnight, spoon out just the set cream on top and proceed as with coconut cream, saving the remaining coconut water for smoothies or other recipes.

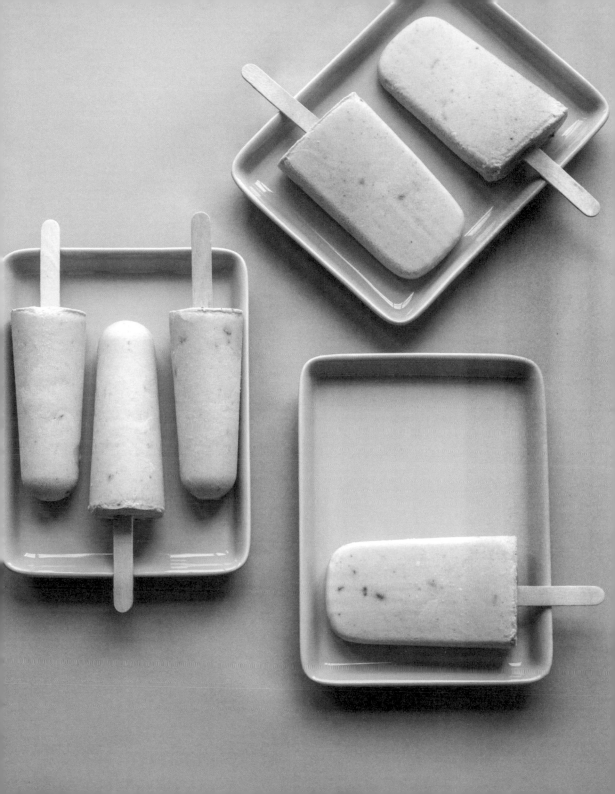

TAHINI TRUFFLES

These truffles are truly addictive — feel free to double or even triple this recipe so you don't run out the same day! They can be kept in the fridge in an airtight container for up to 10 days and in the freezer for up to 2 months.

120 g/1¼ cups dark chocolate 70% cocoa, finely chopped
110 ml/⅓ cup plus 2 tablespoons soy milk
1 tablespoon light muscovado sugar, coconut sugar or xylitol
pinch of salt
1 tablespoon tahini
⅛ teaspoon bourbon vanilla powder
pinch of ground Ceylon cinnamon
cocoa powder, for coating
sea salt flakes, to serve (optional)

MAKES 18 BITE-SIZED TRUFFLES

Place the chopped chocolate in a heatproof bowl. In a small saucepan, whisk together the milk, sugar or xylitol and salt. Bring gently to a simmer, then remove from the heat and pour over the chocolate. Do not whisk, just rotate the bowl to cover the chocolate completely, cover with a lid/plate and leave to stand for 4 minutes. Add the tahini, vanilla powder and cinnamon and whisk gently until glossy. Leave to cool at room temperature for 20 minutes, then refrigerate uncovered for 1–1½ hours.

To make the truffles, remove the chocolate mixture from the fridge and use a 1-tablespoon measuring spoon to scoop out each portion. Use your hands to quickly roll into non-uniform rounds. Place on a plate, refrigerate for 30 minutes, then roll in cocoa powder and sprinkle with salt flakes (if using) to serve.

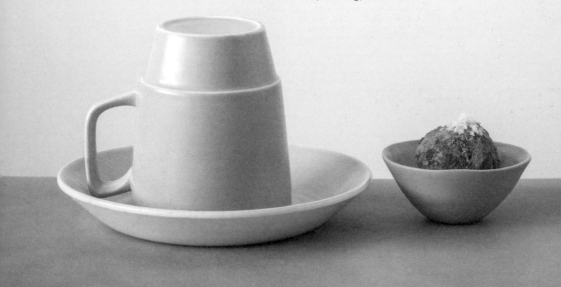

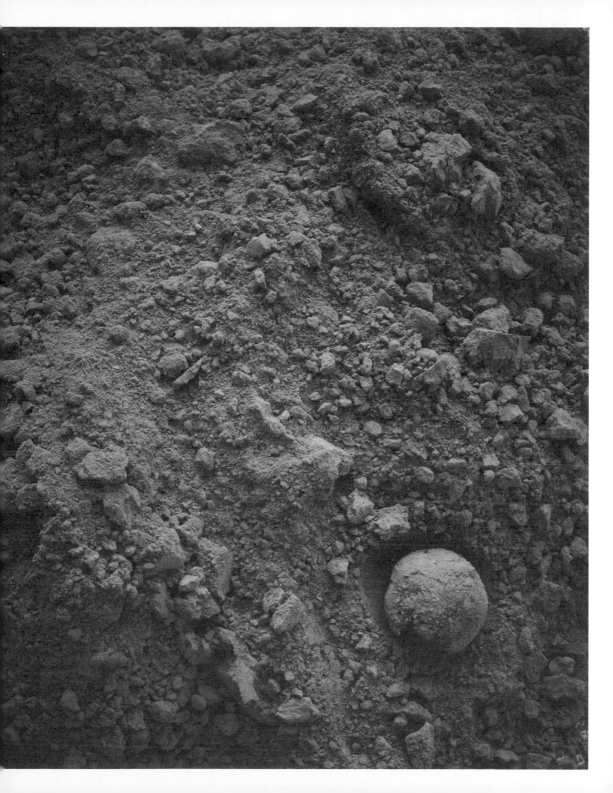

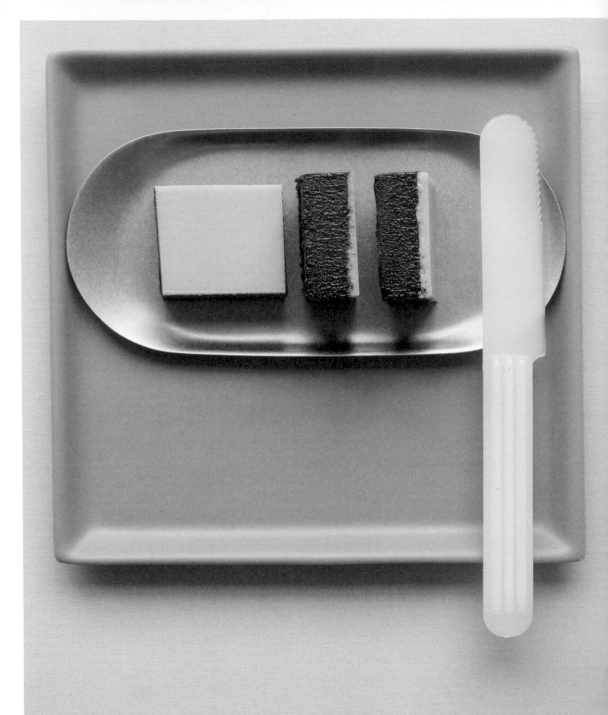

CREAMY DUO FUDGE

In case a sweet treat emergency happens, these fudge bites are the thing to go for! Their rich and creamy taste will stop you buying commercially-produced fudge ever again.

FOR THE BOTTOM LAYER
130 g/½ cup tahini
120 g/1¼ cups dark/bittersweet chocolate 70% cocoa solids
70 g/½ cup coconut sugar
120 ml/½ cup coconut cream
3 tablespoons virgin coconut oil
⅛ teaspoon ground Ceylon cinnamon
⅛ teaspoon fine sea salt

FOR THE TOP LAYER
70 g/½ cup cacao butter
2 tablespoons white tahini
⅛ teaspoon bourbon vanilla powder

18 x 18-cm/7 x 7-inch container, lined with baking parchment

MAKES 36 SQUARES

Place all the bottom layer ingredients in a small saucepan and stir over a very low heat just until the chocolate melts. Pour the mixture into the lined container. Leave to cool and harden, in the fridge or freezer.

Meanwhile, for the top layer, melt the cacao butter in a double-boiler or in a heatproof bowl set over a pan of simmering water, then whisk in the tahini and vanilla powder. Pour over the hardened bottom layer and put back in the fridge/freezer until completely hardened. Lift the baking parchment together with the fudge out of the container, cut into bite-sized pieces and enjoy!

Store leftovers in the fridge in an airtight container for up to 1 week, or in the freezer for up to 2 months.

VARIATION Coconut cream can be substituted with full-fat coconut milk: refrigerate a 400-ml/14-oz. can overnight, spoon out just the set cream on top and proceed as with coconut cream, saving the remaining coconut water for smoothies or other recipes.

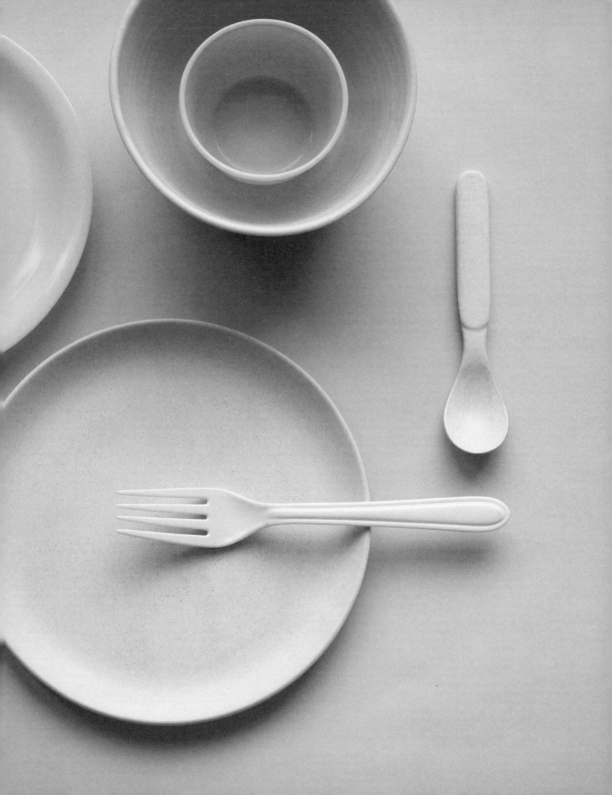

MAINS & SIDES

BEAN & TAHINI BURGERS

Bean and veggie burgers/patties are always satisfying, but adding tahini to the mix does make them more flavourful as well as more nutrient-dense. Couscous can be substituted with leftover brown rice or other grains.

120 ml/½ cup boiling water
100 g/½ cup uncooked couscous
    or 130 g/1 cup pre-soaked
    couscous
260 g/1½ cups cooked borlotti
    beans, well drained
130 g/¾ cup very finely grated
    celeriac/celery root
70 g/½ cup good-quality dried
    breadcrumbs
4 tablespoons tahini
3 tablespoons finely chopped
    onion
2 garlic cloves, crushed
¾ teaspoon salt
½ teaspoon dried pizza seasoning
freshly ground black pepper
sunflower oil or coconut oil
    (melted), for frying

TO SERVE
6 sesame burger/patty buns,
    tahini, lettuce, tomato slices,
    Rich Tahini Coleslaw (see
    page 82), onion slices, Basic
    Tahini Sauce (see page 114)

MAKES 6 LARGE BURGERS/PATTIES

Pour the boiling water over the uncooked couscous, add a little salt, cover and leave to soak for 10 minutes. Or use pre-soaked or leftover couscous.

In a food processor fitted with an 'S' blade, pulse the beans. Transfer to a mixing bowl and add all the remaining ingredients, except the frying oil, but including the couscous. Use your hands to knead the mixture thoroughly – everything should be well incorporated. Chill in the fridge for 20 minutes, or longer. Form into six patties. I usually use a 120 ml/½ cup measuring cup for one burger/patty – fill it and then turn over onto a tray. Pat down to make a nicely shaped burger/patty.

Preheat a cast-iron pan over a medium heat. Pour in 1 tablespoon of oil and add two or three burgers/patties (add more oil and more burgers/patties if your pan is bigger). Fry for about 5 minutes on each side, adding another tablespoon of oil after the flip. When ready, the burgers/patties should be cooked thoroughly, charred a little and forming a thin crust.

For each burger/patty, slice a sesame bun in half and toast. Spread the bottom with tahini, add lettuce (optional) and tomato slices, top with a few tablespoons of coleslaw, add the burger/patty then top with onion slices and a drizzle of basic tahini sauce. Top it off with your toasted top bun and you're all set!

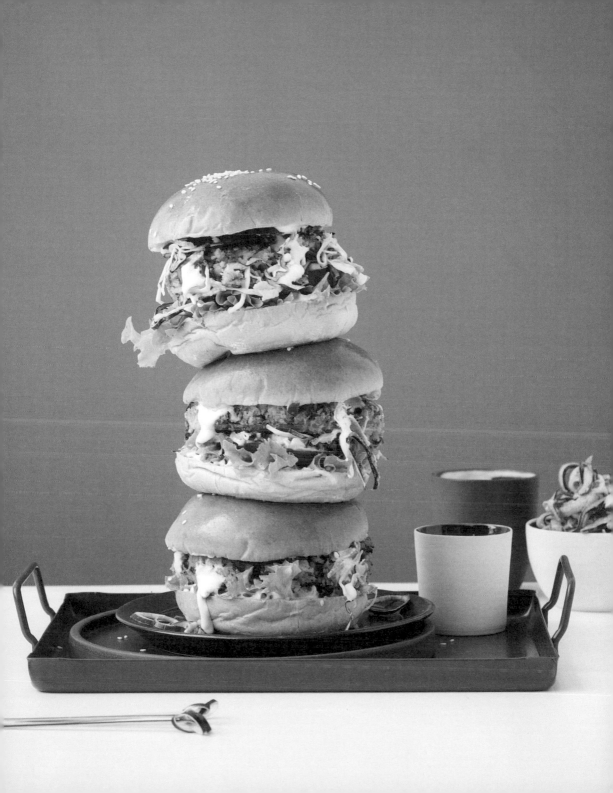

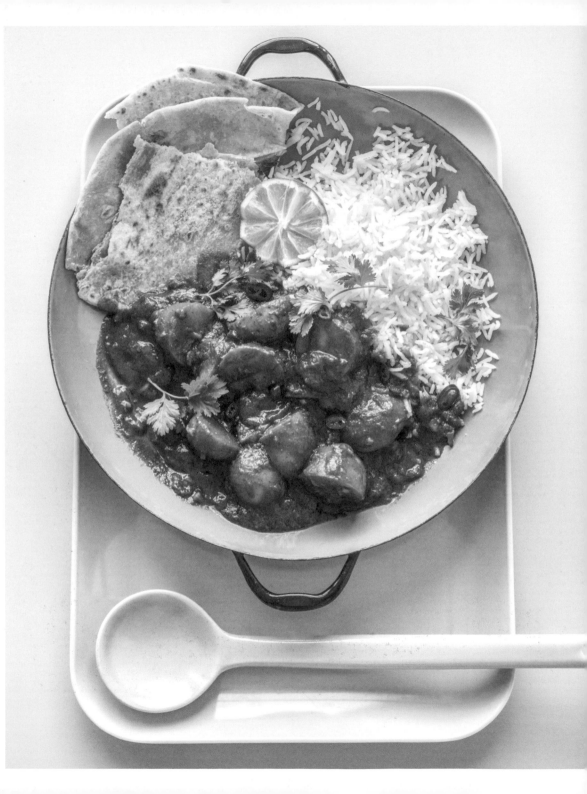

TAHINI & POTATO CURRY

This recipe, like others in the book, avoids added oil and uses tahini instead - it not only adds good fats but also contributes to the creaminess of this curry, so there's no need to use any thickening agents here.

1 large onion, finely chopped
pinch of salt
2-cm/¾-inch piece of fresh ginger, peeled and finely chopped
2 garlic cloves, chopped
1½ tablespoons mild curry powder
2 teaspoons ground ginger
2 teaspoons ground turmeric
2 teaspoons garam masala
1 thinly sliced red chilli/chile or ¼ teaspoon chilli/chili powder, or to taste
2 tablespoons tamari soy sauce
1 large potato, peeled and diced
240 ml/1 cup either tomato sauce or coconut milk
240 ml/1 cup hot water
60 g/¼ cup tahini
sliced spring onion/scallion or freshly chopped coriander/ cilantro and lime half, to serve

SERVES 2

In a large, heavy-bottomed pan, dry-sauté the onion with a pinch of salt until fragrant. Add the ginger, garlic and ground spices, combine and fry for another minute over a low heat. Add the tamari soy sauce and stir. Add the diced potato and enough tomato sauce/coconut milk and hot water to cover. Bring to the boil, then lower the heat and simmer, covered, until the potatoes become soft. Add more liquid during cooking, if necessary.

Stir in the tahini and let the curry boil one last time. Adjust the seasoning, to taste.

Sprinkle with coriander/cilantro and sliced chilli/chile (if using) just before serving. Serve with basmati rice and chapatis or toasted pitta bread, a lime half and a big bowl of salad greens.

SESAME-FULL QUICHE

You can make the pastry in advance and the quiche can be kept in the fridge for a few days – perfect for packed lunches and picnics.

1 onion, chopped
2 garlic cloves, chopped
½ red (bell) pepper, deseeded and cubed
2 tablespoons light sesame oil
1 vegetable stock cube
¼ teaspoon ground turmeric
½ teaspoon smoked paprika
½ teaspoon dried oregano
420 g/2½ cups silken tofu, crumbled
60 g/¼ cup tahini
60 ml/¼ cup soy or oat cream
2 tablespoons nutritional yeast
100 g/1 cup broccoli florets, steamed
2 tablespoons each unhulled sesame seeds and black sesame seeds

FOR THE PASTRY/CRUST

260 g/2 cups unbleached plain/ all-purpose flour
90 g/⅔ cup finely ground yellow cornflour/cornstarch
1½ teaspoons aluminium-free baking powder
salt and ground black pepper
180 g/1½ cups non-hydrogenated margarine
3 tablespoons unhulled sesame seeds
1 tablespoon rice or agave syrup

30-cm/12-inch loose-based tart pan

SERVES 4–6

Preheat the oven to 180°C (350°F) Gas 4.

To make the pastry/crust, combine the flour, cornflour/cornstarch, baking powder and ¼ teaspoon salt in a food processor and pulse to mix. Add the margarine and sesame seeds and pulse 6–8 times, until the mixture resembles coarse meal, with pea-sized pieces of margarine. Add the syrup and 2 tablespoons ice-cold water and pulse again a couple of times. Only if necessary, add more ice-cold water, 1 tablespoon at a time, pulsing until the mixture just begins to clump together. If you pinch some of the crumbly dough and it holds together, it's ready. If the dough doesn't hold together, add a little more water and pulse again. Be careful not to add too much water as this would make the crust tough.

Place the dough in a mound on a clean surface. Work the dough just enough to form a ball; do not over-knead. Form a disc, wrap in clingfilm/plastic wrap and refrigerate for at least 1 hour, or up to 2 days. If you're in a hurry, chill the dough in the freezer for 20 minutes. Roll it out between two pieces of baking parchment about 3 cm/ 1¼ inches wider than the tart pan. Oil the pan. Using a rolling pin, transfer the dough over the pan and press in to cover the entire surface and the sides. Remove excess dough by pressing it outwards with your fingers and patch up any holes with leftover dough. Prick the base all over with a fork and bake in the preheated oven for 8-10 minutes, until just lightly puffed.

To make the filling, sauté the onion, garlic and red (bell) pepper in the sesame oil with a pinch of salt, until

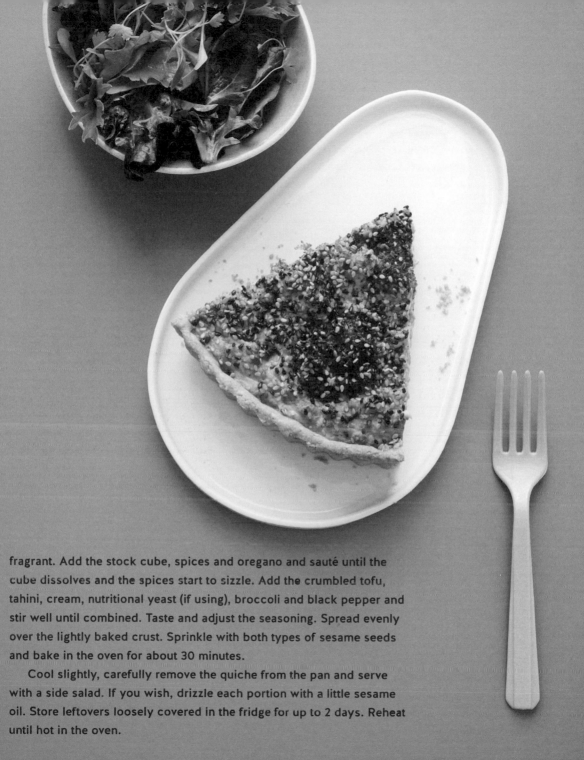

fragrant. Add the stock cube, spices and oregano and sauté until the cube dissolves and the spices start to sizzle. Add the crumbled tofu, tahini, cream, nutritional yeast (if using), broccoli and black pepper and stir well until combined. Taste and adjust the seasoning. Spread evenly over the lightly baked crust. Sprinkle with both types of sesame seeds and bake in the oven for about 30 minutes.

Cool slightly, carefully remove the quiche from the pan and serve with a side salad. If you wish, drizzle each portion with a little sesame oil. Store leftovers loosely covered in the fridge for up to 2 days. Reheat until hot in the oven.

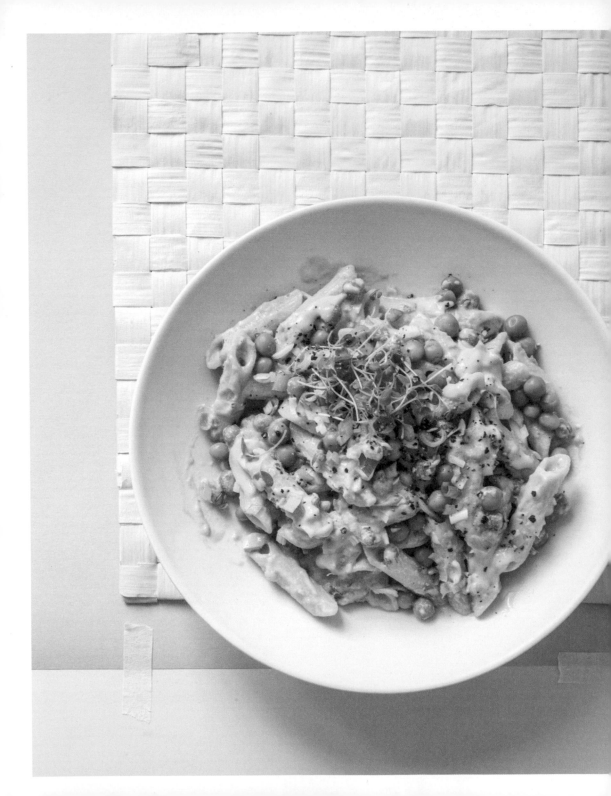

GINGER, PEAS & TAHINI PASTA

I use tahini to make this sauce creamy, and you'll never notice the absence of oil! Tahini is a much more wholesome source of good fats, and oil is overused in cooking anyway, so avoiding it from time to time is actually a good idea.

130 g/1 cup peeled fresh or frozen peas
1 tablespoon very finely chopped (peeled) fresh ginger
2 garlic cloves, finely chopped
2 tablespoons tamari soy sauce, or to taste
4 tablespoons tahini
1 soft pitted date, very finely chopped
240 ml/1 cup oat or soy cream
160 g/2 cups dry gluten-free penne pasta, cooked until al dente
4 spring onions/scallions, finely chopped
salt and crushed black pepper

SERVES 2

Cook the peas in a pan of boiling water until soft but still bright green. Drain and set aside.

Dry-fry the ginger and garlic with a pinch of salt in a frying pan/skillet until fragrant, then add the tamari, tahini, chopped date and cream and bring to the boil, whisking vigorously. Add a little hot water if necessary – the sauce needs to be thick but not sticky.

Pour the sauce over the cooked pasta, season with crushed black pepper, mix well to incorporate, taste and add more tamari/salt if needed. Stir in the peas and spring onions/scallions, leaving some peas and onion greens sauce-free so that the bright green colour stays intact. Serve immediately.

SEED & TAHINI FALAFEL

You'll love this vegetable-rich recipe! It's a raw version of healthier falafel bites that will surprise and impress even the most sceptic eaters. These pink falafel make a perfect lunchbox or picnic item served with any tahini-based sauce and a juicy summer salad of ripe tomatoes, crisp cucumber, leaves and slightly bitter olives. Or, in the winter, pair with a hearty soup for a quick lunch or light dinner.

140 g/1 cup sunflower seeds
  (raw or slightly sprouted)
1 carrot (about 60 g/2¼ oz.)
½ raw beet(root)
  (about 85 g/3 oz.)
40 g/⅓ cup ground flaxseeds/
  linseeds
grated zest of 1 organic orange
1 tablespoon freshly squeezed
  orange juice
2 tablespoons freshly snipped
  chives
¼ teaspoon ground turmeric
¼ teaspoon ground coriander
4 tablespoons tahini
1 teaspoon umeboshi vinegar
  (optional)
salt
1 tablespoon unhulled sesame
  seeds, for sprinkling

*dehydrator lined with a tex-flex
  sheet (or a baking sheet lined
  with baking parchment)*

MAKES 16 SMALL FALAFEL

In a food processor fitted with an 'S' blade, separately chop the sunflower seeds (you want a slightly chunky consistency), then the carrot with the beet(root). Mix together in a bowl, then add the ground flaxseeds/linseeds, orange zest and juice, chives, spices, tahini and vinegar, if using, and combine into a compact paste.

Form into 16 small balls with moist hands, then flatten them slightly. Sprinkle the top of each falafel with unhulled sesame seeds, and place on the lined dehydrator or baking sheet.

Dehydrate on 60°C (140°F) for 1 hour, then lower to 45°C (115°F) and continue dehydrating until the falafel form a crust on the outside, with a still slightly moist inside (this takes 4–5 additional hours). (Alternatively, use the oven: turn it to the lowest setting, and put in the baking sheet with falafel, wedging the door open with a folded tea/dish towel to prevent overheating.)

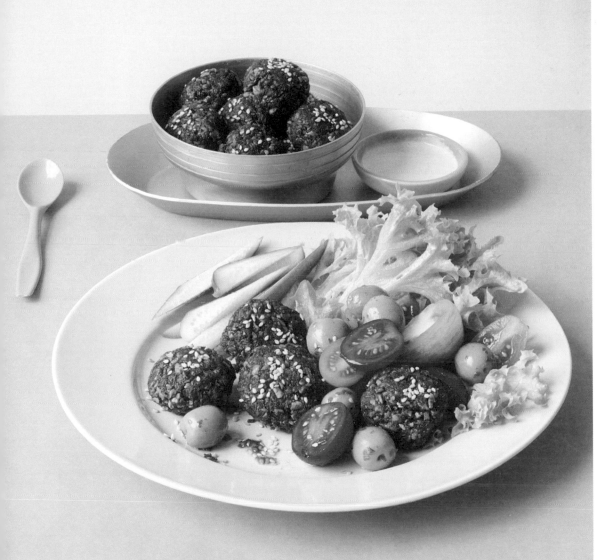

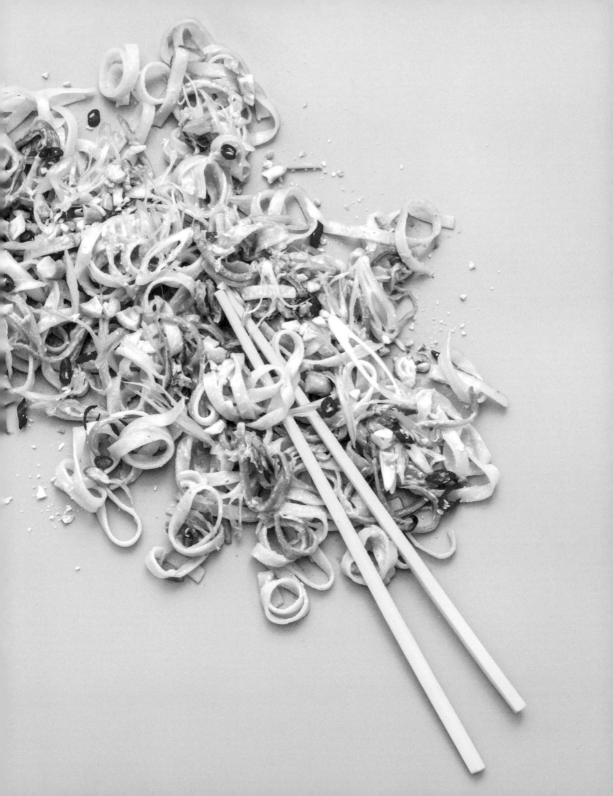

RICE NOODLE PAD THAI

A well-heated cast-iron wok works best for making this simple Pad-Thai: quick-frying should leave the veggies crunchy and the noodles firm but juicy.

1 large onion
2 carrots
175 g/6 oz. dried flat rice noodles (3–5 mm/⅛–¼ inch thick)
tamari soy sauce, to taste
1 vegetable stock cube, or to taste
2 garlic cloves, crushed
1 small fresh red chilli/chile, deseeded and finely chopped, or ¼ teaspoon chilli/chili powder
1 tablespoon agave syrup
2 tablespoons soy or oat cream
4 tablespoons white tahini
salt
4 tablespoons roasted salted cashews, roughly chopped, to serve
coriander/cilantro leaves, (optional)

SERVES 2

Slice the onion into thin half-moons. Cut the carrot into thin matchsticks. Set both aside. Soak/boil the rice noodles according to the packet instructions, then rinse in cold water, drain well and drizzle with a little tamari. Set aside.

In a well-heated wok or a large frying pan/skillet, dry-sauté first the onion with a pinch of salt, then add the carrots and the stock cube and stir until the mixture starts slightly sticking to the wok/pan. Add some tamari, the garlic and the chopped chilli/chile or chilli/chili powder and stir quickly for another minute. Add the syrup, cream, and tahini. Stir and taste. Adjust the thickness by adding a little hot water if necessary and adjust the seasoning to taste – the sauce should be on the saltier side since the noodles are bland.

To serve, place a portion of prepared noodles in the middle of each plate, top with a generous amount of the sauce and sprinkle with chopped cashews and fresh coriander/cilantro, if using.

TAHINI-RICH BUDDHA BOWL

Buddha bowls are big right now, and I totally understand why – it's a plate filled with delicious dishes, combined into a nutritious meal that you can prep in no time! Here's how to make a tahini-rich version.

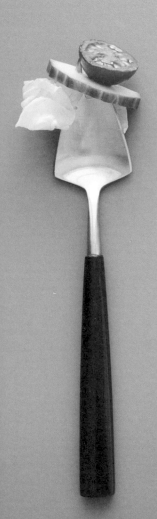

120 ml/½ cup salted boiling water
80 g/½ cup uncooked couscous
80 g/½ cup canned sweetcorn/
   corn kernels, drained and
   rinsed
12 cherry tomatoes, halved
1 medium cucumber, sliced into
   half-moons
8 lettuce leaves, coarsely
   chopped
2 garlic cloves, crushed
2 tablespoons olive oil
2 tablespoons apple cider vinegar
salt
1 x Red Lentil Mash recipe
   (see page 84), to serve
240 ml/1 cup Tahini Gravy
   (see page 120), Ranch Dressing
   or Carrot & Ginger Dressing
   (see page 117)

SERVES 2

Pour the salted boiling water over the couscous in a bowl, cover and steep for 10 minutes. (Or instead of steeping the couscous, you can use any leftover grain you might have sitting in the fridge.)

Mix together all of the ingredients for the salad in a separate bowl.

In two big serving bowls, arrange the couscous, lentil mash and salad. Pour the gravy or dressing of your choice over the couscous and enjoy!

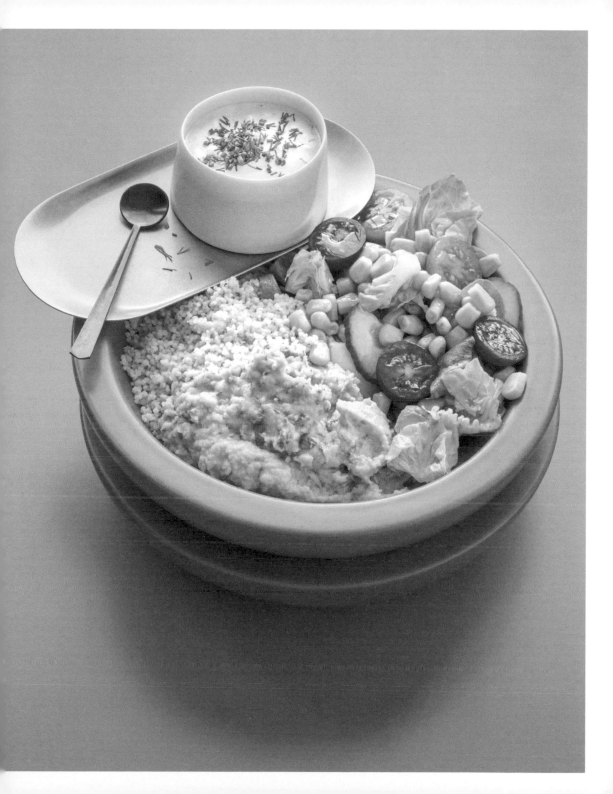

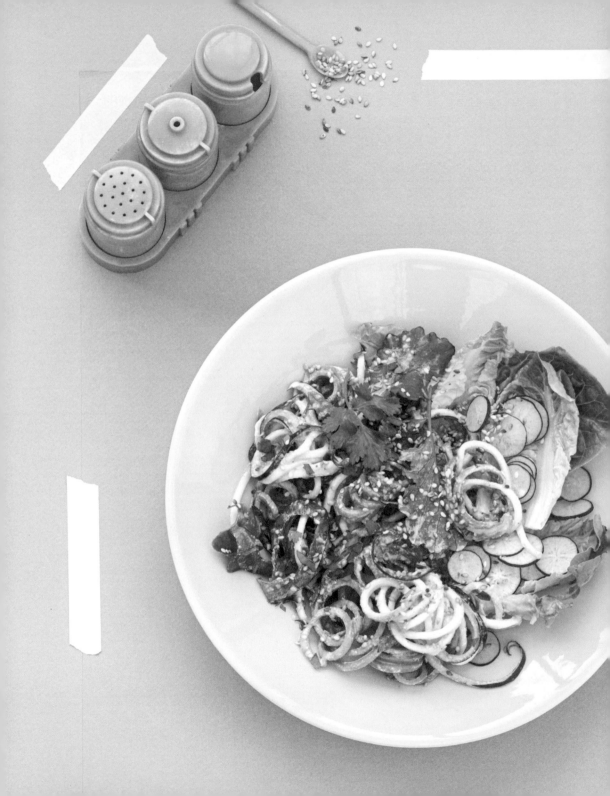

RAW PAD THAI

On hot summer days, this is a nourishing meal that will leave you pleasantly full and save you from standing over the kitchen stove/hob!

1 large carrot
1 medium courgette/zucchini
4 dark kale leaves, stems
    removed, finely chopped
2 spring onions/scallions,
    finely chopped
1 red (bell) pepper, deseeded
    and thinly sliced
crunchy salad leaves, to serve
radish slices, to serve
handful of freshly chopped
    coriander/cilantro or parsley
    leaves, to serve
toasted sesame seeds,
    for sprinkling

FOR THE MARINADE
120 ml/½ cup full-fat coconut
    milk or coconut cream
3 tablespoons white tahini
1 small fresh red chilli/chile,
    deseeded and chopped, or
    ¼ teaspoon chilli/chili powder
1 small piece of fresh ginger
2 garlic cloves, peeled
1 tablespoon tamari soy sauce
2 teaspoons miso paste
1-2 tablespoons freshly squeezed
    lemon juice
1 soft pitted date
1 teaspoon virgin coconut oil,
    melted

SERVES 2

Use a spiralizer to make carrot and courgette/zucchini spaghetti or slice them by hand into long thin matchsticks. Blend all the marinade ingredients together in a blender until smooth and combined, then taste and adjust the seasoning (it should be pretty strong).

Put all the prepared vegetables into a large bowl and pour the marinade over the vegetables, mix well to incorporate and leave to stand for 20 minutes, or longer.

Serve alongside crunchy salad leaves and radish slices with coriander/cilantro or parsley and sesame seeds sprinkled on top.

GRILLED TEMPEH BAGUETTE

I'm a complete fan of tempeh, the fermented soy product rich in protein and full of taste, and I like to use it in veganized versions of hearty meat dishes. In this recipe, to give it even more oomph, thin tempeh slices are marinated in a tahini-enriched marinade and then grilled/broiled – the achieved texture is similar to that of crispy pancetta.

200-g/7-oz. block of tempeh
4 tablespoons tamari soy sauce
3 tablespoons tahini
1 teaspoon smoked paprika
1 teaspoon barbecue spice mix
¼ teaspoon chilli/chili powder
2 tablespoons toasted sesame oil
½ teaspoon garlic powder
¼ teaspoon crushed black pepper

TO SERVE
30-cm/12-inch French baguette
60 ml/¼ cup Tahini & Cashew
  Ranch Dressing (see page 117)
  or vegan mayo
1 ripe avocado
6 big leaves of Romaine lettuce,
  or other greens
9 slices of large ripe tomatoes,
  deseeded
3 tablespoons sauerkraut
  or thinly sliced pickles

*baking sheet lined
  with aluminium foil*

SERVES 3

Preheat the oven to 200°C (400°F) on grill/broiler mode or preheat the grill/broiler to high. Cut the tempeh into slices as thin as possible – depending on the shape of the tempeh block, you should get 20–26 slices. In a bowl, whisk together all the other ingredients to make a smooth marinade.

Place the slices of tempeh on the prepared baking sheet. Cover each slice with the marinade, spreading it to cover the entire slice. Turn them over and do the same on the other side of each slice. Place the baking sheet in the upper part of the oven. Grill/broil for 8–10 minutes, checking occasionally – if you have a powerful oven, the slices could be ready faster. Turn the tempeh slices and grill/broil again until the marinade is soaked in and the slices are crispy and golden brown.

Cut the baguette in half lengthways and lightly toast.

Peel, pit and slice the avocado. Spread some dressing or mayo on both halves of the baguette. Layer the bottom half with slices of tomato and sauerkraut or pickles. Add the tempeh slices, then top with slices of avocado and greens. Cover with the top half of the baguette. Slice across into three same-sized sandwiches with a sharp bread knife and serve immediately. If there are any leftover fillings, serve them on the side.

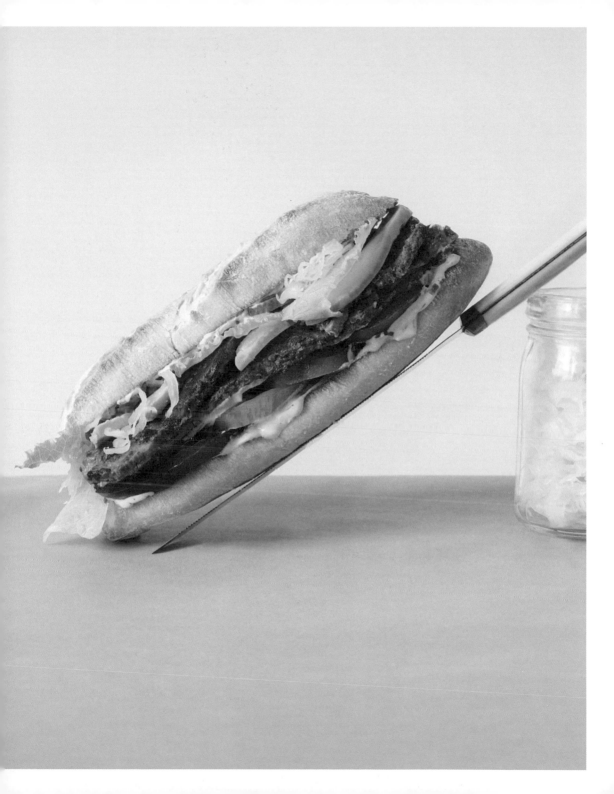

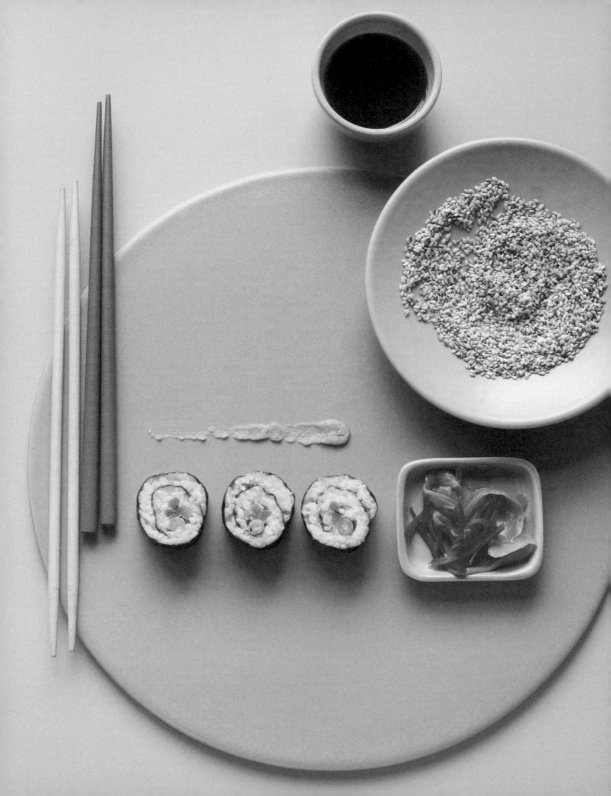

VEGAN SUSHI WITH TAHINI FILLING

There's no reason to think of sushi as a complicated Japanese delicacy that you can't make at home. So here are my instructions to make maki sushi, where the nori is on the outside of the roll, and the filling is inside.

FOR THE SPREAD
4 tablespoons tahini
3 teaspoons umeboshi paste
2 tablespoons dark sesame oil

FOR THE SUSHI
4 toasted nori sheets
475 g/2⅔ cups cooked brown rice or sushi rice
2 medium pickled gherkins, cut lengthways into strips, or other pickled vegetables (sauerkraut, daikon, etc.)
1 carrot, cut lengthways into thin matchsticks
4 spring onion/scallion leaves, washed and drained

FOR THE DIPPING SAUCE
2 tablespoons fresh ginger juice
2 teaspoons tamari soy sauce
2 tablespoons dry-roasted sesame seeds
extra pickles and wasabi paste, to serve

a sushi mat

MAKES 32 PIECES

Prepare the spread by mixing together the tahini, umeboshi paste and sesame oil in a small bowl. The spread is very salty and not meant to be eaten on its own!

Prepare a bowlful of lukewarm water to wet your hands with while making the sushi. Place each nori sheet in turn on a sushi mat, shiny-side down. Wet your hands and spread 120 g/¾ cup of the cooked rice evenly over the nori, except the top side, where you'll want to leave a 1-cm/½-inch margin to make it easier to roll and seal.

To make each maki, spread a heaped tablespoon of the spread across the middle of the rice. Place some gherkin strips, carrot sticks and a spring onion/scallion leaf over the spread, making sure the layer is not thick, as this will make for an overly thick sushi.

Starting from the bottom, roll up the nori and tuck in the vegetables. Continue rolling and press tightly so that the rolled sushi stays sealed. Before serving, slice each sushi into eight same-sized pieces. Repeat the whole process for the other three nori sheets, so you end up with 32 pieces of sushi.

To make the dipping sauce, mix together the ginger juice, tamari and 4 tablespoons of water. Dip a piece of sushi in it, then, before eating, coat it in some sesame seeds.

Serve the sushi with extra pickles and, if you wish, a little wasabi paste, to spice things up!

RICH TAHINI COLESLAW

A fantastic make-ahead salad that should have a place on your menu. We don't eat nearly enough cabbage, especially red cabbage which is pretty cheap and so healthy!

90 g/1½ cups white/green cabbage, shredded
60 g/1 cup red cabbage, shredded
1 large carrot, coarsely grated
1 organic eating apple, cored and cubed
1 onion, finely chopped
2 tablespoons dried cranberries or raisins

FOR THE DRESSING
3-4 tablespoons white tahini
1 tablespoon Dijon mustard
1 tablespoon apple cider vinegar
1 tablespoon umeboshi vinegar
1 garlic clove, crushed
salt, to taste

SERVES 2-4

To make the dressing, whisk or blend all of the ingredients together with 60 ml/¼ cup of water until smooth – it should be runny enough to easily mix with the vegetables. Mix well with the prepared vegetables and fruit and leave to marinate for a couple of hours or refrigerate overnight.

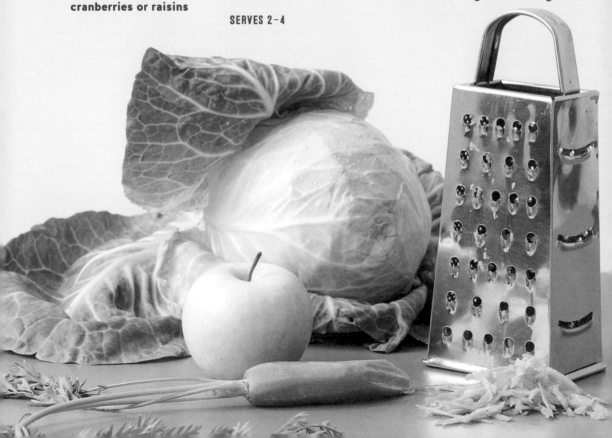

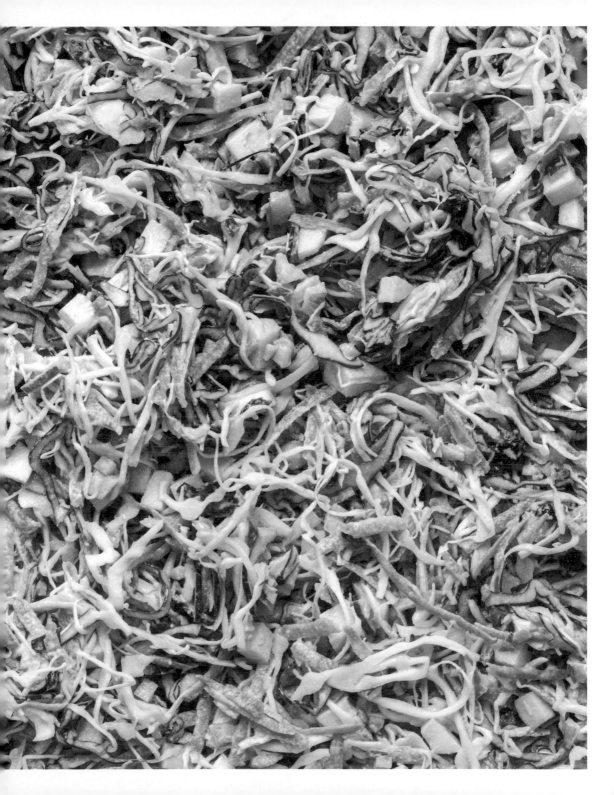

TAHINI-ENRICHED MASH 3 WAYS

Tahini is such a tasty and nutritious addition to purées and mashes made out of different ingredients. Here are my three favourite sides, enriched with sesame paste.

ROOTS & KALE MASH

140 g/2 medium carrots, peeled and chopped
350 g/½ medium swede/rutabaga, peeled
   and chopped
250 g/1 sweet potato, peeled and chopped
180 g/2½ cups kale, middle stems removed
60 g/¼ cup tahini
2 garlic cloves, crushed
salt and freshly ground black pepper
olive oil, for drizzling
toasted sesame seeds, for sprinkling

SERVES 2

Put the carrots, swede/rutabaga and sweet potato into a large pan. Cover with boiling water, add a pinch of salt, bring to the boil, lower the heat and cook, covered, for 10–15 minutes until soft. Add the kale and cook until soft but still bright green. Drain, reserving some of the cooking liquid.

Add the tahini and garlic to the veg in the pan and mash coarsely with a potato masher, adding some reserved cooking liquid as necessary. Add salt and pepper to taste and stir well. Spoon into a serving dish. Drizzle with olive oil and sprinkle with toasted sesame seeds, then serve.

RED LENTIL MASH

180 g/1 cup dried split red lentils
1 bay leaf
60 g/¼ cup tahini
freshly squeezed lemon juice,
   to taste
4 tablespoons freshly chopped
   parsley, chives or coriander/
   cilantro
salt and freshly ground black
   pepper

SERVES 2

Wash and drain the lentils. Fill a heavy-bottomed pan with 480 ml/2 cups water, add the lentils and bay leaf and bring to the boil, uncovered. Lower the heat, half-cover and simmer for 15 minutes, stirring occasionally, until all the water is absorbed and the lentils fall apart. Add a little more hot water during cooking if necessary. Discard the bay leaf. Stir in the tahini and remove from the heat. Add the lemon juice and chopped herbs. Season and serve.

MILLET & CAULI MASH

100 g/½ cup millet
100 g/1½ cups cauliflower florets
¼ teaspoon salt
60 g/¼ cup tahini
hot water, if needed

SERVES 2

Put 480 ml/2 cups water into
a heavy-bottomed pan and
bring to the boil. Add the millet,
cauliflower and salt and bring
back to the boil. Reduce the
heat and simmer, half-covered
for 10 minutes. Stir, cover and
simmer for a further 5 minutes.
Add the tahini and blend into a
purée, adding a little hot water
if needed. Serve immediately.

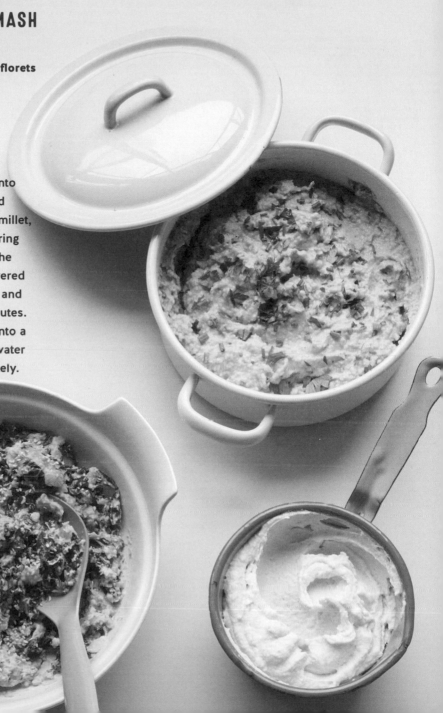

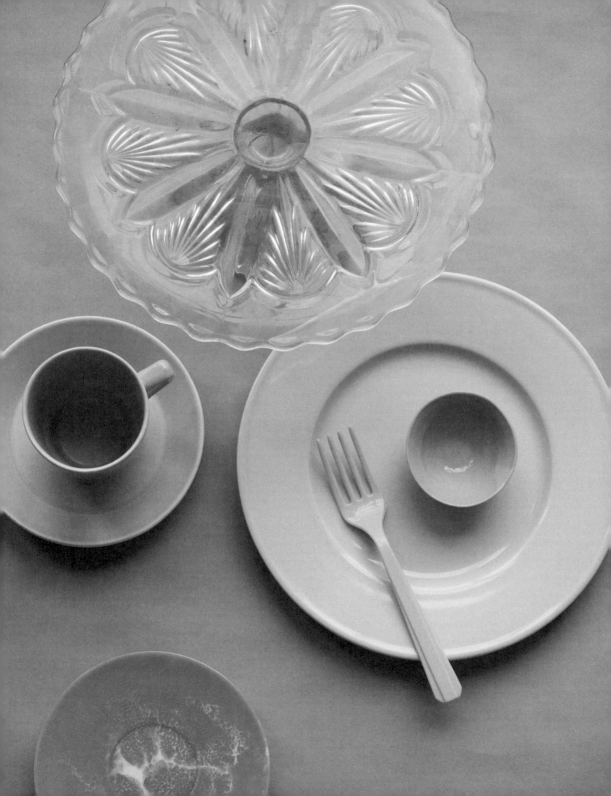

BAKES & DESSERTS

TAHINI BREAD

One of many variations of a simple yeast-free bread I've been making for decades. Instead of the usual addition of oil, I'm adding tahini, and the gram flour makes this bread wonderfully protein-rich.

60 g/¼ cup tahini
240 ml/1 cup sparkling mineral water
240 ml/1 cup kefir or soy yogurt
330 g/2½ cups spelt flour
130 g/1 cup gram flour
2 teaspoons aluminium-free baking powder
1½ teaspoons salt
4 tablespoons raw unhulled sesame seeds, or black, divided

450-g/1-lb. (23 x 12-cm/ 9 x 4½-inch) loaf pan lined with baking parchment (to fit inside without any creases)
oven thermometer (optional)

MAKES ABOUT 14 SLICES

Preheat the oven to 220°C (425°F) Gas 7.

Whisk together the tahini, sparkling water and kefir or soy yogurt in a mixing bowl until dissolved. Sift the flours, baking powder and salt directly into the wet ingredients. Stir vigorously with a spatula until it reaches a smooth, thick batter consistency.

Sprinkle two tablespoons of the sesame seeds onto the bottom of the prepared loaf pan and then spoon in the dough, making sure that it is level. Sprinkle with the remaining sesame seeds and press lightly with your fingers. Put the pan into the preheated oven. Lower the temperature to 200°C (400°F) Gas 6 and bake for 1 hour. Use an oven thermometer if you're not sure about the exact temperature in the oven. If the temperature is below 200°C (400°F) Gas 6, the bread will not rise properly.

Remove the loaf pan from the oven, tip the bread out immediately, peel off the paper and allow to cool completely on a wire rack. This will prevent the bread from absorbing moisture and will keep the crust crisp. Wrap the bread in a clean tea/dish towel and store in a cool, dry place for up to 4 days. Serve in slices.

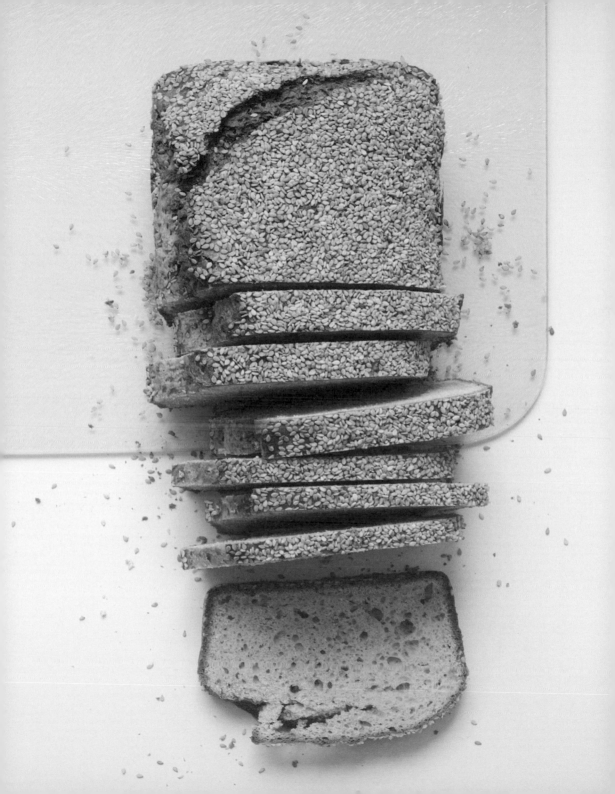

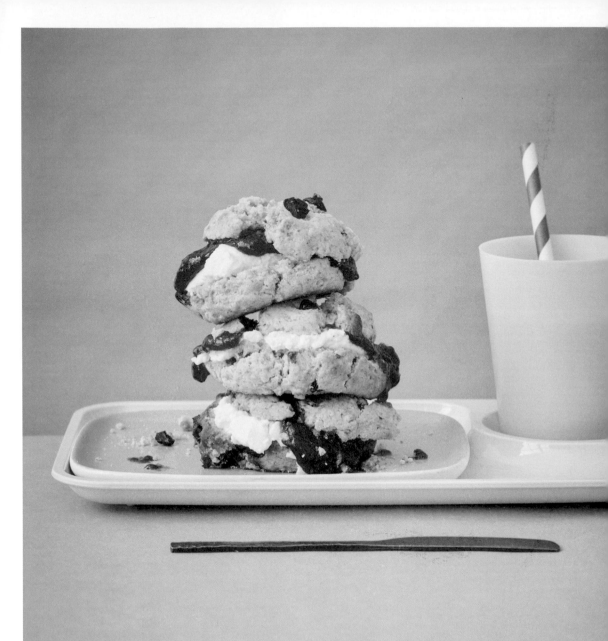

TAHINI MILLET SCONES

These scones taste great served warm, but are also yummy eaten cold, re-heated in the oven, or toasted just before serving.

130 g/1 cup unbleached plain/
  all-purpose flour
70g/½ cup plain wholemeal/
  whole-wheat flour
2 teaspoons baking powder
½ teaspoon salt
60 ml/¼ cup virgin coconut oil,
  melted
5 tablespoons pre-cooked millet
120 ml/½ cup buttermilk (or
  a mixture of soy milk and
  ½ teaspoon vinegar)
3 tablespoons tahini
30 g/¼ cup dried fruit (raisins,
  pitted chopped dates, etc.)
3 tablespoons brown rice or
  agave syrup
jam/preserves of your choice,
  to serve (optional)
whipped soy or oat cream of
  your choice, to serve (optional)

*baking sheet lined with baking
  parchment*

MAKES 10 SCONES

Preheat the oven to 200°C (400°F) Gas 6.

Sift the flours, baking powder and salt into a large bowl. Add the melted coconut oil and stir gently until the mixture resembles fine breadcrumbs. Stir in the millet. Combine the buttermilk, tahini, dried fruit and syrup in a small bowl, then add to the large bowl of other ingredients. Mix briefly with a spatula to form a soft dough.

Scoop ten spoonfuls of dough onto the prepared baking sheet, leaving a little space between the scones (each scone should weigh about 55 g/2 oz.).

Bake in the preheated oven for 15–20 minutes or until risen and golden. Remove from the oven and serve warm with jam/preserves and cream, if desired.

TAHINI & RAISIN MINI MUFFINS

These cuties are rich in fruit and winter spices. They will warm you up and satisfy your sweet cravings after a hearty winter meal.

2 rosehip tea bags
120 g/1 cup raisins
160 ml/⅔ cup boiling water
grated zest and freshly squeezed
   juice of 1 orange
70 g/¼ cup tahini
60 ml/¼ cup date syrup
130 g/1 cup unbleached plain/
   all-purpose flour
1 teaspoon aluminium-free baking
   powder
½ teaspoon bicarbonate of/
   baking soda
¼ teaspoon salt
½ teaspoon ground Ceylon
   cinnamon
¼ teaspoon freshly grated nutmeg
¼ teaspoon ground ginger
60 g/½ cup walnuts, toasted
   and chopped, plus extra for
   topping

24-cup mini muffin pan,
   lined with muffin cases

MAKES 24 MINI MUFFINS

Preheat the oven to 180°C (350°F) Gas 4.

Put the tea bags and raisins into a large heatproof bowl and cover with the boiling water. Leave to steep for 10 minutes. Squeeze and remove the tea bags. Add the orange zest and juice, tahini and date syrup and whisk well to incorporate.

Sift the flour with the baking powder, bicarbonate of/ baking soda, salt and spices into the bowl, then fold into the liquid and gently stir into a smooth batter. Add the nuts and stir well.

Divide the batter evenly between the prepared muffin cups, scatter over the remaining walnuts and bake in the preheated oven for 15–20 minutes or until golden brown on the edges. Remove from the oven and leave to cool in the pan for 10 minutes, then gently remove from the pan and serve warm or cold. Store in an airtight container for 2–3 days.

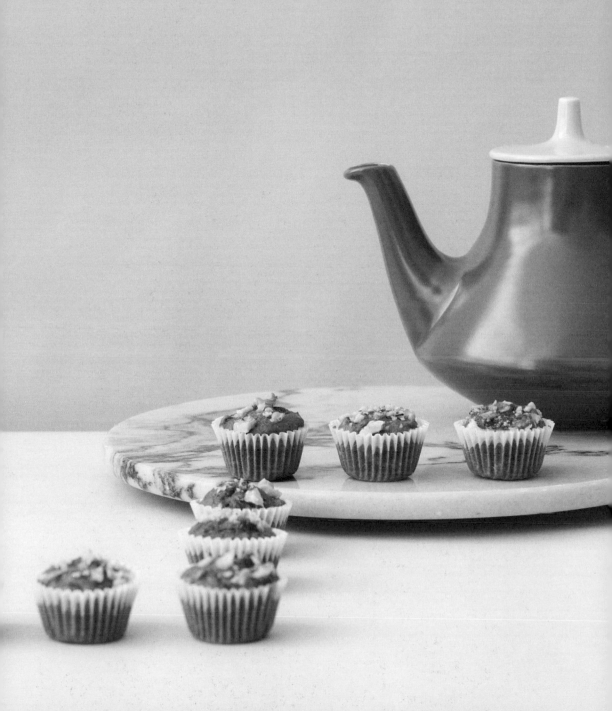

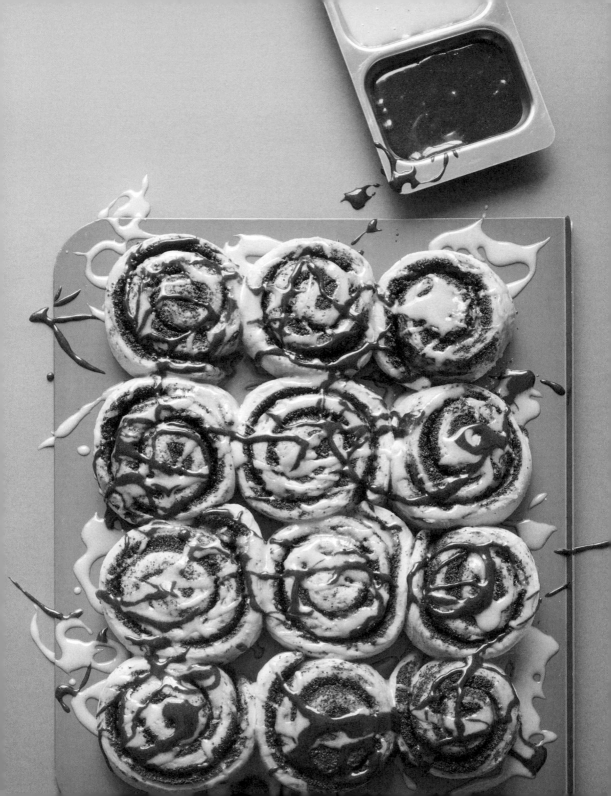

BLACK TAHINI & POPPY SEED SWIRLS

The traditional walnut/hazelnut filling has been substituted with the darker poppy and sesame combo, a must-try!

240 ml/1 cup soy milk
3 tablespoons virgin coconut oil, plus extra for oiling the dough
9 g/1 sachet dried active yeast
1 tablespoon coconut sugar
½ teaspoon salt
390 g/3 cups unbleached plain/all-purpose flour, plus extra for dusting

FOR THE DARK ICING
140 g/¾ cup coconut sugar
2 tablespoons arrowroot powder
2 tablespoons black tahini
coconut or soy milk, if needed

FOR THE LIGHT ICING
260 g/1¼ cups demerara/turbinado or unrefined brown sugar, ground into a powder
2 tablespoons white tahini
1–2 tablespoons soy or coconut milk

FOR THE FILLING
90 g/⅔ cup coconut sugar
1 teaspoon ground Ceylon cinnamon
100 g/1 cup ground poppy seeds
2 tablespoons virgin coconut oil, melted
2 tablespoons black tahini

23 x 30-cm/9 x 12-inch baking pan lined with baking parchment

MAKES 12 SWIRLS

Heat the soy milk and coconut oil in a non-stick pan over a low heat until the oil is dissolved. Leave to cool slightly then add the yeast, coconut sugar and salt and whisk well. Transfer to a large bowl and, using a wooden spoon, mix in the flour. Place on a clean, lightly floured surface and knead for a couple of minutes.

Oil a large bowl and the dough. Put the dough in the bowl, cover with a wet tea/dish towel and leave to rise for 1 hour until doubled in size.

Preheat the oven to 180°C (350°F) Gas 4.

Meanwhile, prepare the icings. In two separate bowls, whisk together the ingredients for the dark icing and the light icing until thick. Set aside.

When the dough is ready, place it between two sheets of baking parchment and use a rolling pin to roll it into a rectangular shape about 5 mm/⅝ inch thick.

To make the filling, combine the sugar, cinnamon and ground poppy seeds in a bowl. Brush the surface of the dough with the melted coconut oil, spread with the tahini and sprinkle the poppy seed mixture evenly over the top.

Gently roll the dough away from you into a log, starting from the longer side of the rectangle. Using a serrated knife, cut the log across into 12 equal rolls. Carefully put the rolls into the prepared baking pan, leaving space between each one. Leave to rise for a further 10–20 minutes, then bake in the preheated oven for 25–30 minutes. Remove from the oven and drizzle with the icings while still hot. Serve.

SESAME CUPCAKES WITH FROSTING

Here's another delicious idea for how to incorporate tahini and sesame seeds into your desserts or bakes!

60 ml/¼ cup aquafaba, chilled
¾ teaspoon aluminium-free
  baking powder, divided
60 ml/¼ cup coconut oil, melted
130 g/⅔ cups coconut sugar
240 ml/1 cup soy milk
1 teaspoon apple cider vinegar
130 g/1 cup Bob's Red Mill
  gluten-free 1-to-1 baking flour,
  or unbleached all-purpose flour
100 g/¾ cup spelt flour or plain/
  all-purpose wholemeal/whole-
  wheat flour
2 tablespoons cocoa powder
½ teaspoon bicarbonate of/
  baking soda
¼ teaspoon salt
50 g/¼ cup sesame seeds,
  toasted and crushed

FOR THE FROSTING
140 g/1 cup non-hydrogenated
  organic margarine
130 g/⅔ cup demerara/turbinado
  sugar or xylitol, ground into
  a fine powder
¼ teaspoon bourbon vanilla powder
60 g/¼ cup tahini
2 tablespoons toasted black
  or unhulled sesame seeds,
  for sprinkling
12-cup muffin pan, oiled
piping/pastry bag fitted with
  a star-shaped nozzle/tip

MAKES 12

Preheat the oven to 180°C (350°F) Gas 4.

For the cupcakes, using a stand mixer, whisk the chilled aquafaba with ¼ teaspoon of the baking powder until stiff peaks form.

In a separate bowl, whisk together the melted coconut oil, coconut sugar, soy milk and vinegar. Sift the dry ingredients (except the sesame seeds, but including the remaining baking powder) directly into the wet mixture and whisk gently until well combined. Add the toasted and crushed sesame seeds and whisked aquafaba and gently fold in.

Spoon the batter into the prepared muffin pan, dividing it equally between the cups. Bake in the preheated oven for 20 minutes. Leave to cool slightly in the pan, then gently remove from the pan and allow to cool completely on a wire rack.

With a sharp knife, carve out a walnut-sized piece of muffin from the top of each one.

To make the frosting, beat the margarine in a stand mixer until fluffy, sift in the sugar and vanilla powders and mix well until smooth. Add the tahini and mix again until velvety. Spoon into the piping/pastry bag fitted with an open star-shaped nozzle/tip and generously frost each cupcake. Sprinkle with toasted sesame seeds and serve.

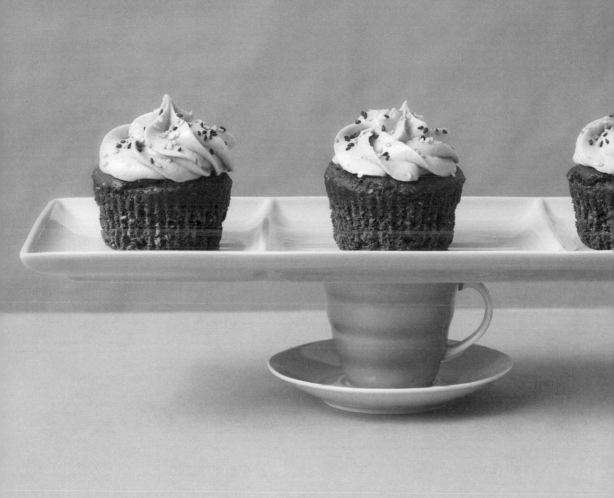

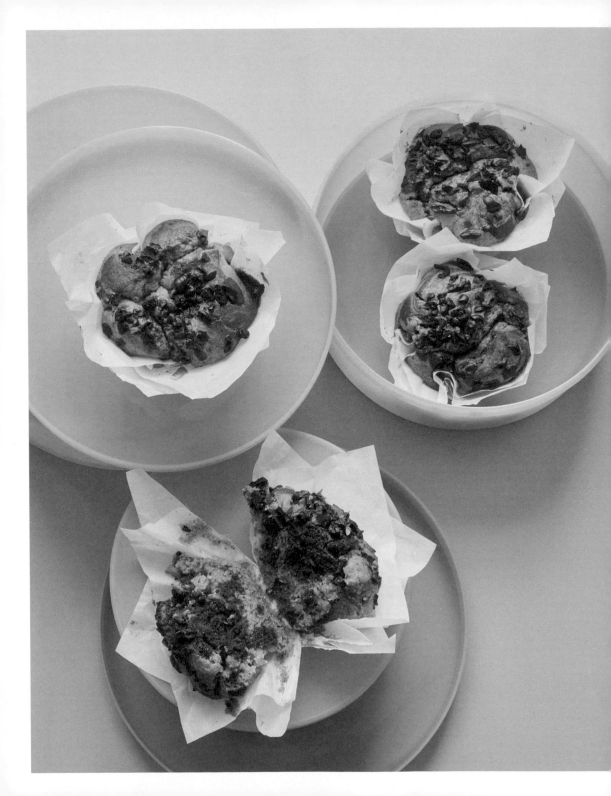

MARBLED MUFFINS

Marble cake, marble squares, marble bundt cake – it seems everyone I know has their own special recipe for this delicious cake creation. So, I made myself a promise that one day I, too, would have my own special marbled baked recipe! And here it is, in the shape of these wonderfully moist, banana-cocoa-tahini flavoured marbled muffins.

70 g/¼ cup tahini
1 ripe banana, peeled
60 ml/¼ cup virgin coconut oil, melted
300 ml/1¼ cups coconut milk
1½ teaspoons apple cider vinegar
160 ml/⅔ cup pure maple syrup
¼ teaspoon pure almond extract (optional)
130 g/1 cup unbleached plain/all-purpose flour
60 g/½ cup plain/all-purpose wholemeal/whole-wheat flour
¼ teaspoon bourbon vanilla powder
1 teaspoon baking powder
½ teaspoon bicarbonate of/baking soda
¼ teaspoon salt
grated zest of 1 lemon
1 tablespoon raw cocoa nibs, plus extra for sprinkling
1 tablespoon raw cocoa powder

12-cup muffin pan lined with squares of baking parchment

MAKES 10–12

Preheat the oven to 180°C (350°F) Gas 4.

Blend the tahini and banana together with the liquid ingredients in a blender until smooth. Sift the flours, baking powder, bicarbonate of/baking soda, vanilla powder and salt directly into the wet ingredients. Add the lemon zest. Whisk gently until you have a smooth batter.

Spoon one-third of the mixture into a separate bowl and fold in the cocoa nibs and cocoa powder.

Divide the plain muffin mixture between 10–12 lined muffin cups. Put a spoonful of the cocoa mixture on top of that and, with the help of a chopstick or skewer, mix in a little to get a marbled pattern. Sprinkle with the extra cocoa nibs.

Bake in the preheated oven for 18–20 minutes. Remove from the muffin pan and allow to cool on a wire rack. This is a great picnic and lunchbox muffin!

JAM-FILLED TAHINI COOKIES

When making these cookies, I recommend putting the jam/preserves onto the cookies after baking. It's far less mess and means that the jam/preserves won't run over the edges and burn, as it often does if cookies are filled before baking.

120 ml/½ cup rice or agave syrup
60 g/¼ cup virgin coconut oil (melted), or sunflower oil
80 g/⅓ cup tahini
soy milk, if needed
130 g/1 cup unbleached spelt or wheat flour
¼ teaspoon Ceylon cinnamon
¼ teaspoon salt
100 g/1 cup rolled oats, ground into fine flour
50 g/½ cup sesame seeds, toasted and ground into flour

FOR THE FILLING
110 g/4 tablespoons plum, apricot or strawberry jam/preserves (or use more than one flavour)
2 teaspoons rum or water

baking sheet lined with parchment paper

MAKES 32 COOKIES

Preheat the oven to 180°C (350°F) Gas 4.

Whisk the liquid ingredients with the tahini in a mixing bowl, then sift in the flour, cinnamon and salt. Whisk again to incorporate, then add the rolled oats, oat flour and ground sesame seeds. Mix well with a spatula into a thick dough. If too dry, add a little soy milk.

Shape the dough into small, walnut-sized balls, place on the baking sheet then use a small, sharp knife to carve a little hole in the top of each one, about the size of ¼ teaspoon. Bake the cookie balls in the preheated oven for 15 minutes until lightly golden, then remove from the oven.

For the filling, in a small saucepan whisk together the jam/preserves and rum or water and heat until boiling.

Carefully fill each hole in the hot cookies with the hot jam/preserves. Leave to cool before serving. The cookies can be stored in an airtight container for up to a week.

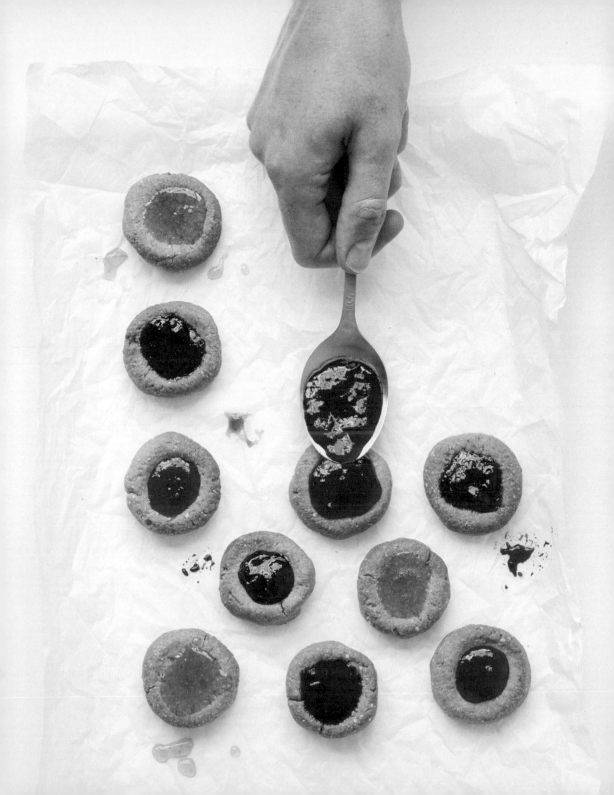

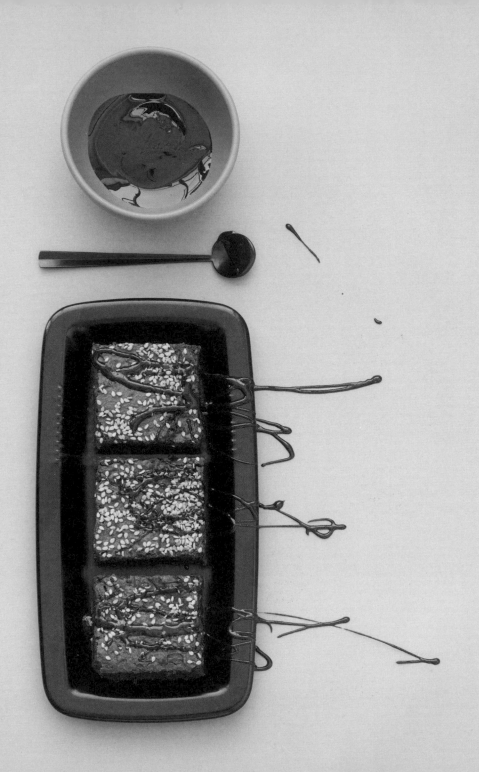

SESAME BROWNIES

Blended beans and tahini give a wonderful texture to these brownies and it's a great way to introduce plant protein and calcium to kids!

200 g/1½ cups finely chopped dark/bittersweet chocolate 70% cocoa
300 g/2 cups canned (drained and rinsed) unsalted chickpeas or haricot/navy beans
60 ml/¼ cup virgin coconut oil, melted
240 ml/1 cup brown rice or pure maple syrup
grated zest and freshly squeezed juice of 1 lemon
130 g/½ cup tahini
80 g/⅔ cup unbleached plain/ all-purpose flour
40 g/⅓ cup plain all-purpose wholemeal/ whole-wheat flour
1 tablespoon baking powder
¼ teaspoon salt
¼ teaspoon ground Ceylon cinnamon
4 tablespoons unhulled sesame seeds, for sprinkling
2 tablespoons melted chocolate, for serving

23 x 30-cm/9 x 12-inch baking pan, oiled

MAKES ABOUT 20

Preheat the oven to 180°C (350°F) Gas 4.

Melt the chocolate in a heatproof bowl set over a saucepan of simmering water, making sure that the base of the bowl does not touch the water.

Put the melted chocolate, chickpeas or haricot/navy beans, melted coconut oil, syrup, lemon zest and juice and tahini in a food processor and blend until smooth.

Mix the flours, baking powder, salt and cinnamon together in a mixing bowl. Add the bean mixture and fold in with a spatula until smooth.

Spoon the cake mixture into the prepared baking pan and spread evenly with a spatula. Sprinkle with the sesame seeds.

Bake in the preheated oven for 20 minutes. Do not overbake – they are supposed to be a little gooey! Allow to cool completely in the baking pan. Cut into squares to serve drizzled with melted chocolate. Alternatively, I like to serve them with a little homemade apricot jam/ preserves which contrasts beautifully with the rich, heavy chocolate of these brownies.

OAT & TAHINI CAKE WITH CHIA JAM

This gluten-free granola-like cake can be cut into bars and enjoyed for breakfast, as a snack or even for dessert.

300 g/3 cups rolled oats, ground into a coarse flour
25 g/¼ cup fine rolled oats
130 g/1 cup Bob's Red Mill 1-to-1 gluten-free mix
1 teaspoon ground Ceylon cinnamon
1 teaspoon aluminium-free baking powder
¼ teaspoon bourbon vanilla powder
¼ teaspoon salt
160 ml/⅔ cup agave, rice or maple syrup
170 g/⅔ cup tahini
soy milk, if needed

FOR THE CHIA JAM/PRESERVES
200 g/1 cup fresh or frozen (thawed) raspberries
2 tablespoons agave, rice or maple syrup
1 teaspoon freshly squeezed lemon juice
1 tablespoon chia seeds

baking sheet lined with baking parchment

MAKES 12 BARS

Preheat the oven to 180°C (350°F) Gas 4.

To make the chia jam/preserves, put the raspberries into a pan and bring to a quick boil. Add the remaining ingredients then reduce the heat and simmer. Blend into a smooth jam/preserves in a blender, and set aside.

To make the cake, put all of the dry ingredients into a large bowl and whisk together. In a separate bowl, whisk the syrup and tahini together, then add to the dry ingredients. Stir well, adding a little soy milk if the mixture is too dry.

Divide the dough in half. With slightly wet hands, spread one half of the dough onto the prepared baking sheet. Evenly spread the chia jam/preserves over the bottom crust, then crumble the remaining dough over the jam/preserves and press down with moist hands or a metal spatula to even out the top layer.

Bake in the preheated oven for 25 minutes or until the mixture is golden. Leave to cool in the baking sheet before slicing into bars. This cake will keep for up to a week, wrapped in a tea/dish towel.

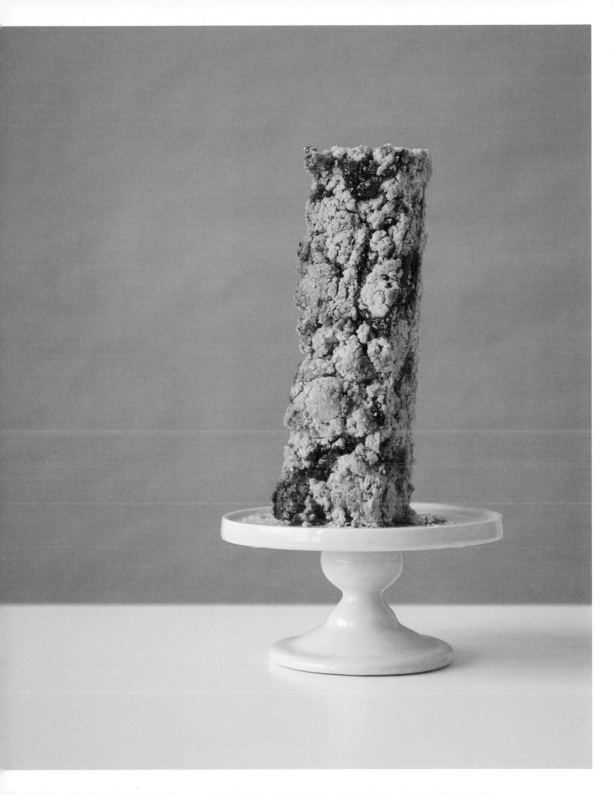

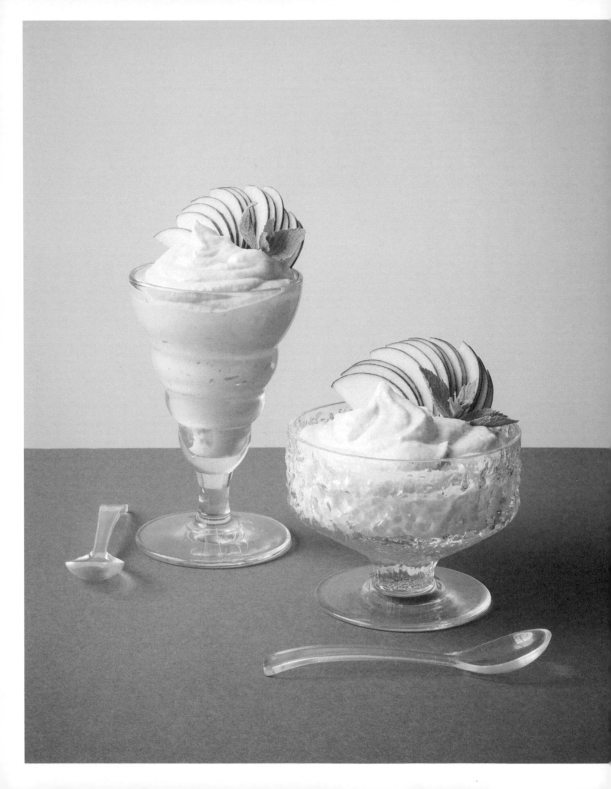

CREAMY APPLE SAUCE DESSERT

I love sweet treats, but I am also aware that it's not a good idea to eat baked cakes or chocolate every single day, even if made with healthier ingredients. This is one of the ultra-healthy dessert options if you want to avoid gluten and any added sugar and still get your daily sweet fix!

480 ml/2 cups apple sauce
80 g/½ cup unsalted cashews, soaked in cold water for 4 hours, rinsed and drained
4 tablespoons white tahini
4 soft pitted dates, or to taste
¼ teaspoon ground Ceylon cinnamon, plus extra to serve
pinch of salt
½ small red eating apple, sliced into thin half-moons, to serve
mint or melissa sprigs, to serve

SERVES 2

Blend all of the ingredients together in a blender until creamy, gradually adding a little warm water to reach the desired consistency.

Divide between two dessert bowls and serve warm, or chilled. Decorate with fresh apple slices, mint or lemon balm/melissa sprigs and dust with cinnamon.

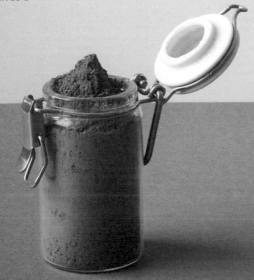

TAHINI SANDWICH COOKIES

These tahini cookies work well on their own, but filling them with chocolate and turning the plain cookies into creamy sandwich cookies is quite fun and they are also very yummy to bite into, so why not?

120 ml/½ cup rice, agave or maple syrup
3 tablespoons soy milk, or as needed
80 g/⅓ cup tahini
130 g/1 cup unbleached plain/all-purpose flour
40 g/¼ cup plain wholemeal/whole-wheat flour
¼ teaspoon bicarbonate of/baking soda
⅛ teaspoon salt
10 g/1 sachet bourbon vanilla sugar
80 g/⅓ cup powdered demerara/turbinado sugar

FOR THE FILLING
120 g/1¼ cups dark/bittersweet chocolate 70% cocoa solids, broken into small pieces
60 ml/¼ cup soy or oat cream
2 tablespoons powdered demerara/turbinado sugar

baking sheet lined with baking parchment

FOR 14 SANDWICH COOKIES

Preheat the oven to 180°C (350°F) Gas 4.

Put all of the wet ingredients into a large bowl. Whisk well, then sift in all of the dry ingredients. Combine into a smooth dough, adding a little extra soy milk if too dry, or a little extra flour, if too sticky.

Tip the dough out onto a clean surface and knead into a ball. Wrap in clingfilm/plastic wrap and rest in the fridge for at least 30 minutes, or overnight.

Remove the dough from the clingfilm/plastic wrap and place between two sheets of baking parchment, then use a rolling pin to roll into a rectangle approximately 2–3 mm/¹⁄₁₆–⅛ inch thick. Use a knife to trim the edges and cut rectangle-shaped cookies about 3 x 5 cm/1¼ x 2 inches. Knead the off-cuts of dough into a new ball and repeat the rolling and cutting process until you have 28 cookies. Transfer to the prepared baking sheet and bake in the preheated oven for 10 minutes or until lightly golden. Slide the baking parchment with the cookies from the baking sheet onto a wire rack to cool.

While the cookies are cooling, make the filling. In a double boiler, melt the chocolate then add the cream and whisk until smooth. Refrigerate until thick enough for spreading. Spread the filling onto the flat sides of 14 cookies. Top with the remaining cookies and refrigerate until firm. Serve chilled or at room temperature. Store in an airtight container for up to a week.

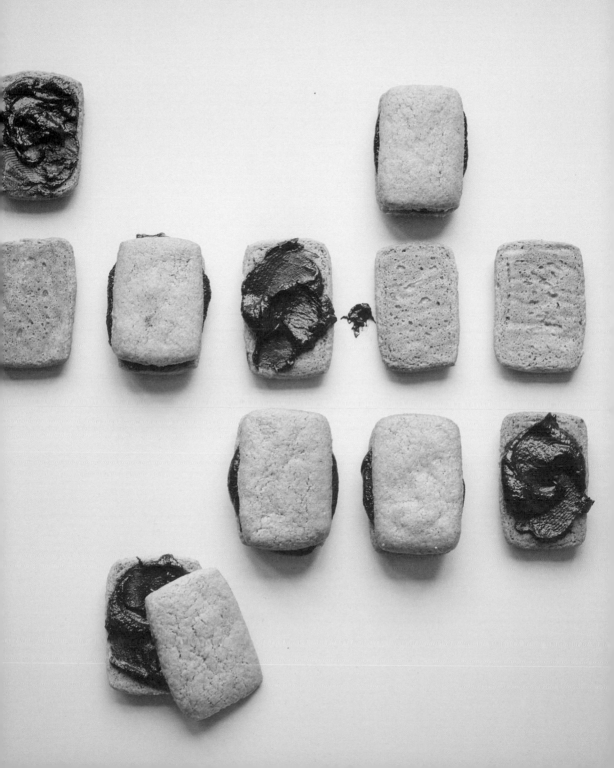

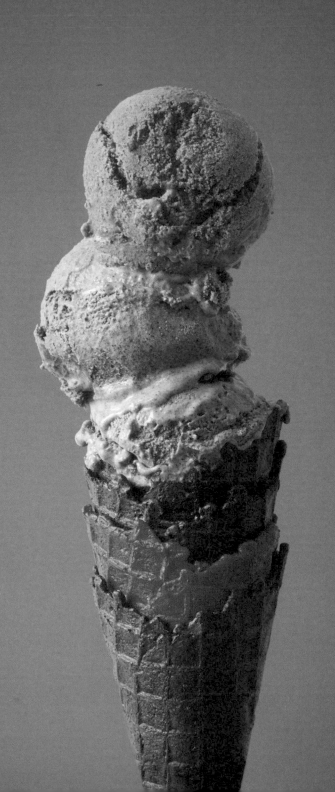

BLACK TAHINI & COCONUT ICE CREAM

An interesting looking & tasting ice cream: coconut, tahini, vanilla... what's there not to like?

130 g/½ cup black tahini
400-ml/14-oz. can coconut cream
240 ml/1 cup soy or oat cream
80 ml/⅓ cup maple syrup or other liquid sweetener
3 tablespoons arrowroot powder
¼ teaspoon bourbon vanilla powder
4 ice-cream cones, to serve
2 tablespoons large coconut flakes, to serve

ice-cream maker (optional)

SERVES 4

Blend all of the ingredients except the coconut flakes and cones into a creamy paste in a bowl. Place into the ice-cream maker (if using) and follow the instructions.

To make without the ice-cream maker, pour the mixture into a deep, wide freezerproof container and place in the freezer for 45 minutes. Remove from the freezer and stir vigorously to break up any frozen crystals. Return to the freezer and repeat the stirring process every 30 minutes for 2–3 hours. When ready, scoop the ice cream into ice-cream cones, sprinkle with coconut flakes and serve immediately, or transfer the ice cream to a covered airtight or freezerproof container until ready to serve. The ice cream can be stored in the freezer for up to 1 month.

VARIATION Substitute the coconut cream with full-fat coconut milk. Refrigerate two 400-ml/14-oz. cans over-night, spoon out just the cream on top and proceed as with coconut cream, reserving the remaining coconut water for smoothies or other recipes.

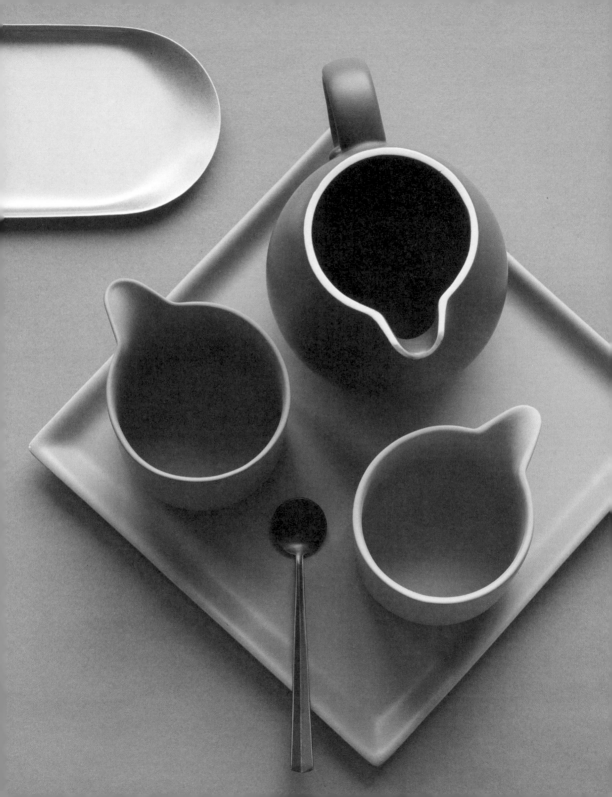

SAUCES & DRESSINGS

BASIC TAHINI SAUCE

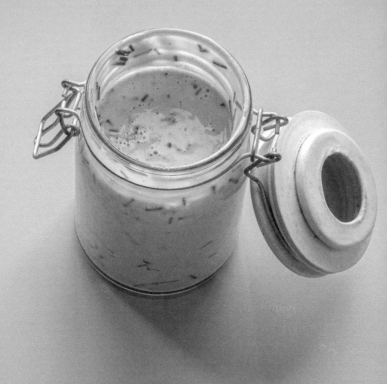

Simple, creamy
and nutritious!

4 tablespoons tahini
1 garlic clove, crushed
1 tablespoon freshly chopped
  chives
about 120 ml/½ cup oat, rice
  or almond milk
freshly squeezed lemon juice,
  to taste
salt and freshly ground black
  pepper

MAKES ABOUT 150 ML/²/₃ CUP

Mix together the tahini, crushed
garlic and chopped chives in a
bowl or jar and add just enough
milk to form a smooth sauce.
Add a little lemon juice and
salt and pepper to taste. Cover
and store in the fridge for up to
3 days.

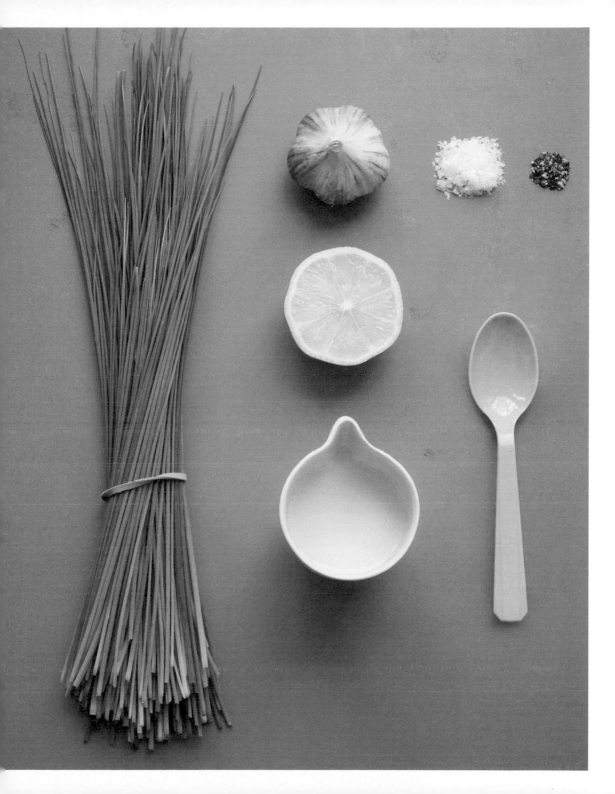

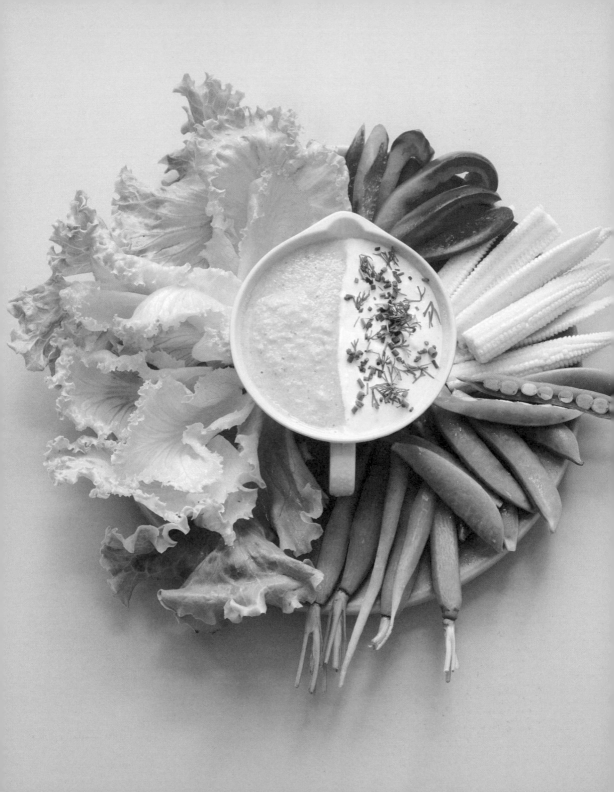

TAHINI & CASHEW RANCH DRESSING

Try this vegan alternative to a regular ranch dressing. It can be used not only for dressing salads but also as a dip for crudités or as a spread in sandwiches.

130 g/½ cup tahini
60 g/½ cup cashews, soaked in cold water for 4 hours, drained and rinsed
130 g/½ cup vegan mayonnaise
2 tablespoons apple cider vinegar, or to taste
2 garlic cloves, peeled
1 tablespoon Dijon mustard
½ teaspoon salt
10 g/¼ cup freshly chopped dill and chives, plus extra to serve
freshly ground black pepper

MAKES 320 ML/1⅓ CUPS

Using a blender, blend the tahini, cashews, mayonnaise, vinegar, garlic, mustard and salt, slowly adding cold water to reach the desired consistency. Transfer to a bowl and fold in the chopped herbs and pepper to taste. Taste and adjust the vinegar and/or salt, to taste. Cover and keep refrigerated for up to 4 days.

CARROT & GINGER DRESSING

An interesting combo of tastes: pungent ginger, sweet carrot and slightly bitter tahini.

100 g/1 large carrot, chopped
70 g/1 small onion, chopped
2-cm/¾-inch piece of fresh ginger, peeled
2 tablespoons parsley greens
2 soft dates, pitted
2 tablespoons tahini
2 tablespoons soy or oat cream
1 tablespoon umeboshi vinegar or salt to taste
1 tablespoon apple cider vinegar, or to taste

MAKES 320 ML/1⅓ CUPS

Using a blender, blend all the ingredients together with 120 ml/½ cup cold water into a smooth dressing. Store in a sealed jar in the fridge for up to a week.

SIMPLE TAHINI VINAIGRETTE

A simple dressing with the addition of tahini that can be made ahead and stored in a sealed jar in the fridge for a couple of days.

4 tablespoons tahini
12 tablespoons apple cider
   vinegar, or to taste
grated zest and freshly
   squeezed juice of 2 lemons
4 tablespoons tamari soy sauce
15 g/½ cup finely chopped
   parsley greens
water, as needed
salt and freshly ground black
   pepper

MAKES 415–480 ML/1¾–2 CUPS

Whisk all the ingredients together in a bowl until the tahini is dissolved. Taste and adjust the seasoning. It should taste quite strong and a bit on the salty side to complement the mild taste of raw salad and vegetables.

ANTI-FATIGUE DRESSING

Umeboshi is a Japanese pickled plum that is an effective digestive aid as it helps combat nausea and fatigue.

6 tablespoons tahini
2–3 tablespoons umeboshi paste
4 tablespoons soy or oat cream,
   or more
freshly squeezed lemon juice,
   to taste

MAKES ABOUT 240 ML/1 CUP

Mix all the ingredients into a paste in a small bowl. This can be used as a salad dressing (add more cream to make it runny), as a dip for raw veggies or as a spread.

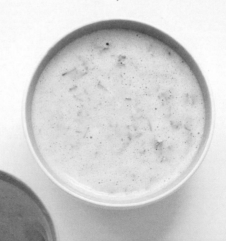

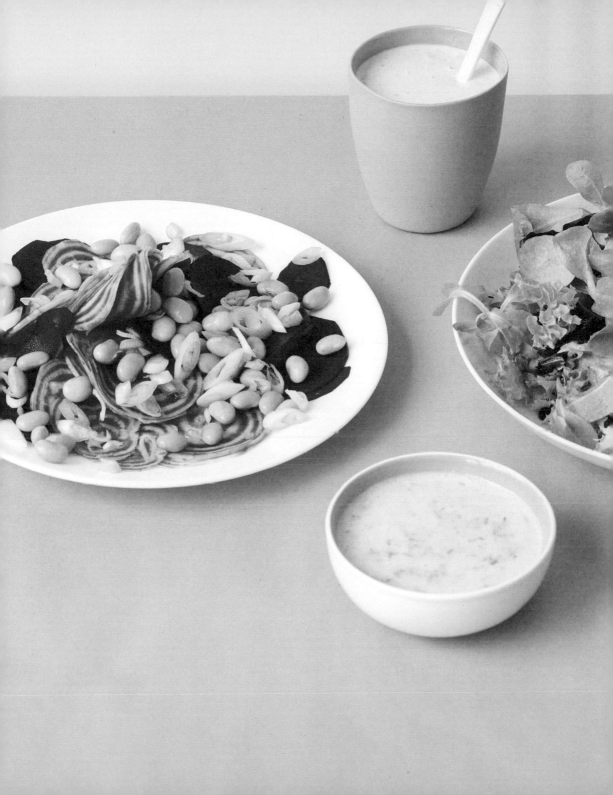

WHITE MISO & WHITE TAHINI GRAVY

A very quick and simple recipe to make when you feel you need to juice up your meal! This gravy tastes great poured over cooked or raw vegetables or a burger/patty.

90 g/¾ cup onion, sliced into thin half-moons
4 tablespoons light sesame oil
4 garlic cloves, crushed (optional)
1 teaspoon apple cider vinegar
1 teaspoon rice or agave syrup
2 tablespoons unbleached plain all-purpose flour (or kuzu, cornflour/starch or arrowroot powder paste)
4 tablespoons white tahini
2 tablespoon white miso paste (shiro miso)
2 teaspoons Dijon mustard (optional)
salt and crushed black pepper

MAKES ABOUT 480 ML/2 CUPS

In a large frying pan/skillet sauté the onion in the oil with a pinch of salt over a low heat until translucent and soft. Add the garlic (if using) and cook until fragrant. Slightly increase the heat and add salt to taste, the vinegar and syrup and stir well until it sizzles. Slowly add the flour (or paste), whisking vigorously for a minute, then, still whisking, add 235 ml/1 cup cold water little by little, until smooth. Add the tahini, white miso, mustard (if using) and pepper, then taste and add more salt if needed. Store in the fridge for up to 3 days.

VARIATION Sauté 25 g/½ cup chopped fresh mushrooms or 2 tablespoons soaked, drained and chopped dried mushrooms with the onion for extra flavour.

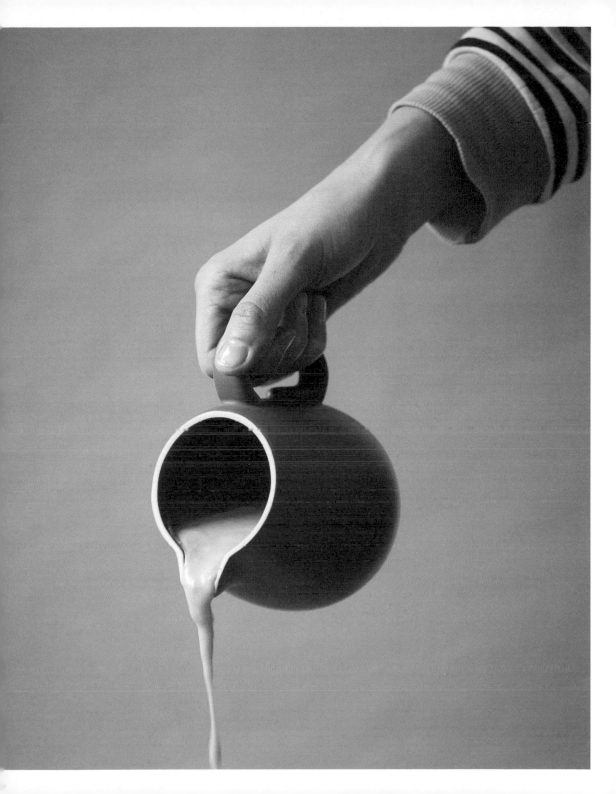

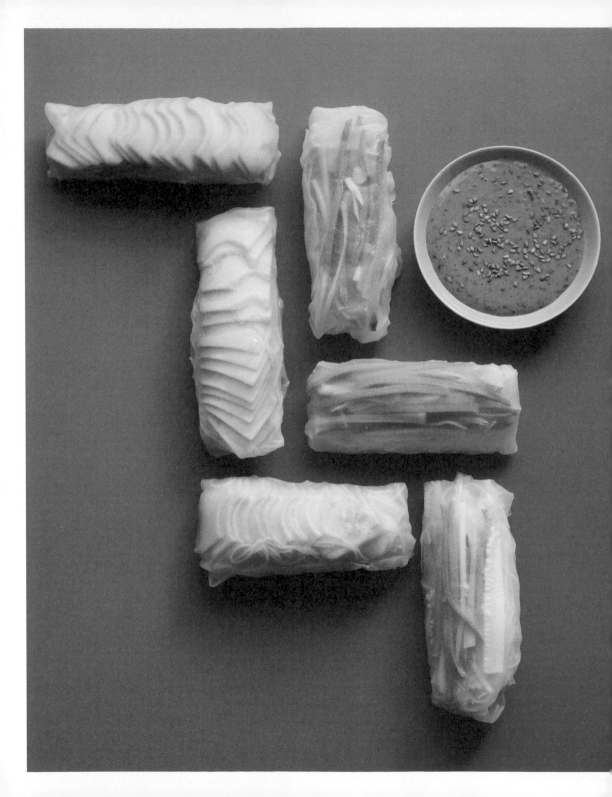

SWEET & SOUR SAUCE

This is my go-to dipping sauce
for rice paper spring rolls. So yum!

2 tablespoons tahini
2 tablespoons apple cider vinegar
1 tablespoon tamari soy sauce
1 tablespoon agave syrup or
    1 soft date, pitted and finely
    chopped
½ teaspoon chilli/chili powder,
    or to taste
1–2 tablespoons warm water
2 tablespoons toasted sesame
    seeds, for sprinkling (optional)

MAKES ABOUT 120 ML/½ CUP

Whisk all the ingredients except
the sesame seeds together in a
small bowl. Gradually add the
warm water if needed, to reach
the desired consistency. Sprinkle
with toasted sesame seeds
and serve as a dipping sauce
to accompany your favourite
savoury snack.

AVOCADO & TAHINI PASTA SAUCE

If you ask me, any dish with avocado is delicious and when you add tahini to it, the nutritional value just goes up and up! This creamy sauce goes amazingly well with a good-quality spelt or rice spaghetti. It will only take a couple of minutes to prepare and will make you happy and satisfied for much longer!

2 ripe avocados
4 tablespoons tahini
2 tablespoons olive oil
2 tablespoons umeboshi vinegar
   (or tamari soy sauce or salt,
   to taste)
175 g/6 oz. dried spelt or rice
   spaghetti, cooked until
   al dente and drained
handful of garlic sprouts,
   or other seed sprouts
2 tablespoons toasted black
   sesame seeds, to garnish

SERVES 2

Peel, halve and stone/pit the avocados, then blend along with the tahini, olive oil and umeboshi vinegar (or soy sauce/salt) in a food processor or a blender until smooth. Add a little cold water if it's very thick. Taste and adjust the seasoning, bearing in mind that it should be on the saltier side, since pasta needs a strong sauce.

Pour the sauce over the hot spaghetti and mix thoroughly. Serve immediately, sprinkling each portion with half of the garlic sprouts (or other sprouts) and a tablespoon of black sesame seeds.

VARIATION You can use any nut or seed butter instead of tahini; peanut butter, for example, makes a nice sauce, too! You can basically make endless variations of this sauce, adding garlic, onion, freshly squeezed lemon juice or crushed black pepper, all depending on what you have in your fridge or cupboard. Bon appétit!

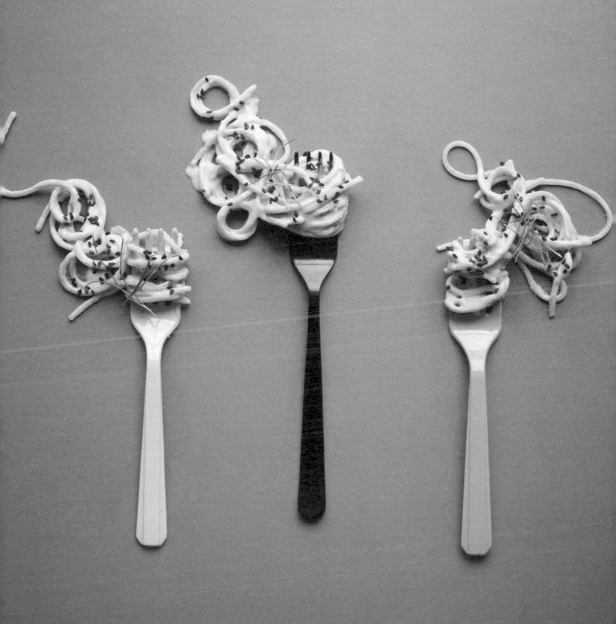

INDEX

ACKNOWLEDGEMENTS

As in all my cookbooks, I'd like to thank my family, friends and especially people who follow my work for their support, enthusiasm and trust. I get e-mails and messages from people all over the world on a weekly basis, letting me know that they are using my recipes and how much some things I have written and shared changed their diet for the better. I get photos of my recipes done by others all the time too – it's such a good feeling knowing my books aren't just a decoration on the kitchen shelves. Instead, they are actually being used and that is what keeps me motivated to continue with what I'm doing!

I'd also like to thank the whole RPS team, above all Julia Charles for her support over the years, and Alice Sambrook and Miriam Catley for their expertise, patience and flexibility with deadlines! Thank you to Megan Smith for her beautiful design work and the photography team, Clare Winfield, Emily Kydd and Alexander Breeze. I'm so grateful to be surrounded by such a creative and supportive team.

Finally, I'd like to thank you for choosing this book as your cooking companion! It will bring tasty and nourishing dishes to your family table, and I hope you will feel the pinch of passion secretly added to each and every one of the recipes I shared in this cookbook – that tiny ingredient can make a gigantic difference, bringing back joy into your daily life!

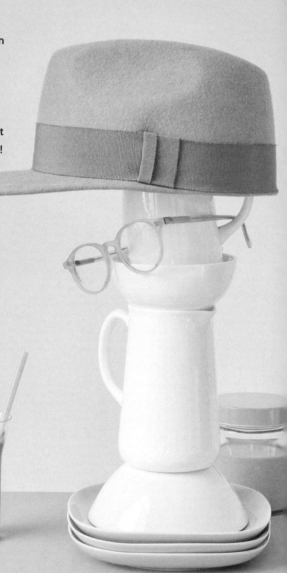

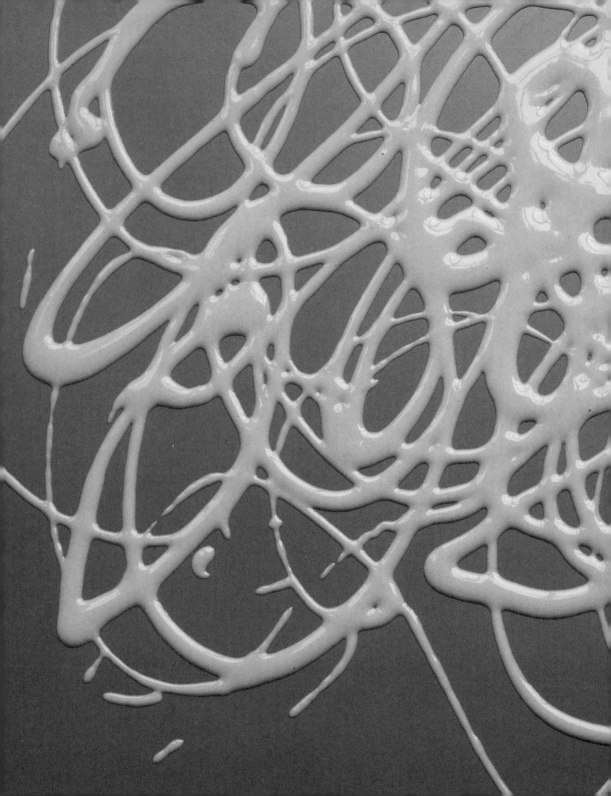